State of Art
in
Ophthalmic
Surgery

Basic to Advance

to

I owe my ophthalmic career to the wonderful institution of Dr Rajendra Prasad Center for Ophthalmic Science, at All India Institute of Medical Sciences (AIIMS), New Delhi and dedicate this video atlas of ophthalmic surgery to everyone who has worked to make this centre what it is and also my consultants at Sydney Eye Hospital, University of Sydney, Sydney, Australia who taught lovingly and gave a much needed different perspective to an Indian student. Also I owe a lot to our patients who trust us and believe in us, as well as my family—husband (Dr Suresh K Pandey), parents (Group Captain KM Sharma & Smt Sudha Sharma) and daughter (Ishita), for being so supportive.

Vidushi Sharma

My career in ophthalmology was greatly influenced by some of the best known teachers and pioneers in ophthalmology. I would like to dedicate this video atlas of ophthalmic surgery to my teachers and pioneers in ophthalmology—Professor Amod Gupta (PGIMER, Chandigarh), Professor Jagat Ram (PGIMER, Chandigarh), Professor Amar Agarwal (Chennai), Dr. Mahipal S Sachdev (New Delhi), Late Prof David J. Apple (USA), Professor Frank A Billson (Australia), Dr. E. John Milverton (Australia), and Dr Anthony J Maloof (Australia), who have inspired and motivated me to strive for excellence and achieve greater heights each day. We have no identity without our patients who trust us and believe in us, as well as my family —wife (Dr Vidushi Sharma), parents (Shri Kameshwar P Pandey and Smt Maya Pandey) and daughter (Ishita), for being so supportive.

Suresh K Pandey

CBS Surgical Video Series in Ophthalmology

State of Art
in
Ophthalmic
Surgery

Basic to Advance

Editors

Vidushi Sharma
MD (AIIMS, New Delhi), FRCS (UK)

Suresh K Pandey
MS (PGIMER, Chandigarh), ASF (USA)

SuVi Eye Institute and Lasik Laser Centre
C13 Talwandi, Kota, Rajasthan, India

Visiting Assistant Professor
John A Moran Eye Center, University of Utah
Salt Lake City, Utah, USA
and
Sydney Eye Hospital, Save Sight Institute
University of Sydney, Sydney, Australia

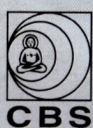

CBS

CBS Publishers & Distributors Pvt Ltd

New Delhi • Bengaluru • Chennai • Kochi • Mumbai • Pune
Hyderabad • Kolkata • Nagpur • Patna • Vijayawada

State of Art in
Ophthalmic Surgery
Basic to Advance

ISBN: 978-81-239-2459-5

First Edition: 2014

Published by Satish Kumar Jain for

CBS Publishers & Distributors Pvt Ltd
4819/XI Prahlad Street, 24 Ansari Road, Daryaganj, New Delhi 110 002, India.
Ph: 23289259, 23266861, 23266867   Website: www.cbspd.com
Fax: 011-23243014   e-mail: delhi@cbspd.com; cbspubs@airtelmail.in

Corporate Office: 204 FIE, Industrial Area, Patparganj, Delhi 110 092
Ph: 4934 4934   Fax: 4934 4935   e-mail: publishing@cbspd.com; publicity@cbspd.com

Branches

- **Bengaluru:** Seema House 2975, 17th Cross, K.R. Road, Banasankari 2nd Stage, Bengaluru 560 070, Karnataka
  Ph: +91-80-26771678/79   Fax: +91-80-26771680   e-mail: bangalore@cbspd.com
- **Chennai:** 20, West Park Road, Shenoy Nagar, Chennai 600 030, Tamil Nadu
  Ph: +91-44-26260666, 26208620   Fax: +91-44-42032115   e-mail: chennai@cbspd.com
- **Kochi:** 36/14 Kalluvilakam, Lissie Hospital Road, Kochi 682 018, Kerala
  Ph: +91-484-4059061-65   Fax: +91-484-4059065   e-mail: kochi@cbspd.com
- **Mumbai:** 83-C, Dr E Moses Road, Worli, Mumbai 400018, Maharashtra
  Ph: +91-22-24902340/41   Fax: +91-22-24902342   e-mail: mumbai@cbspd.com
- **Pune:** Bhuruk Prestige, Sr. No. 52/12/2+1+3/2 Narhe, Haveli (Near Katraj-Dehu Road Bypass), Pune 411 041, Maharashtra
  Ph: +91-20-64704058, 64704059, 32342277   Fax: +91-20-24300160   e-mail: pune@cbspd.com

Representatives

- **Hyderabad** 0-9885175004 • **Kolkata** 0-9831437309, 0-9051152362
- **Nagpur** 0-9021734563 • **Patna** 0-9334159340   • **Vijayawada** 0-9000660880

Printed at: HT Media Ltd., Noida

Preface

This video atlas **State of Art in Ophthalmic Surgery** covers the basic techniques, and major surgical techniques in phacoemulsification, premium IOLs (multifocal, toric and multifocal toric) pterygium, glaucoma and oculoplastic surgery. A total of 65 videos cover the majority of the commonly performed ophthalmic surgeries. A unique feature of this video atlas is inclusion of presentations discussing ophthalmic practice management and career options for young ophthalmologists.

We believe video atlas will be helpful of ophthalmologists worldwide. Our sincere thanks to Mr SK Jain, Mr YN Arjuna, Mr Dinesh Dheek and Ms Ritu Chawla of CBSP&D, New Delhi, India, for their valuable help in bringing out and publishing this project.

Vidushi Sharma
Suresh K Pandey

E-mail: suvieye@gmail.com,
Website: www.suvieye.com

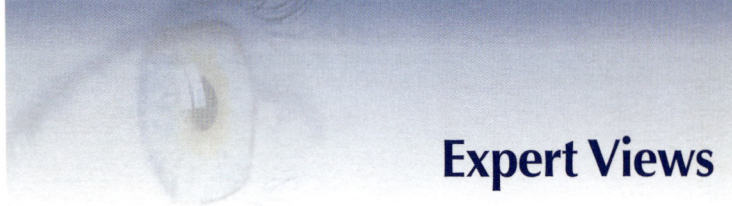

Expert Views

State of Art in Ophthalmic Surgery is a very interesting series of surgical videos compiled by Dr Vidushi Sharma and Dr Suresh K Pandey, alumni of Sydney Eye Hospital, Save Sight Institute, Sydney, Australia. A total of 65 videos in 4 DVD will be really helpful for ophthalmology residents as well as practicing ophthalmologists to get an idea about the various ophthalmic surgeries. Most of the videos are accompanied by an excellent narration covering the finer

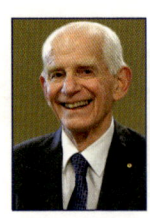

points of the surgeries. I really liked the presentations on career options for young ophthalmologists and changing trends in ophthalmic practice. I congratulate Dr Suresh and Dr Vidushi for their sincere efforts to bring out *State of Art in Ophthalmic Surgery*.

Professor Frank A Billson
Professor of Ophthalmology University of Sydney
Director of Sight Foundation Microsurgical Skills Centre
Sydney Eye Hospital
8 Macquarie St Sydney NSW 2000, Australia

I congratulate Dr Vidushi Sharma, and Dr Suresh K Pandey for bringing out video atlas *State of Art in Ophthalmic Surgery* containing a variety of ophthalmic surgeries. Almost all the commonly performed surgeries are well covered and the videos are of very good quality. The section on ophthalmic practice management and career options for young ophthalmologists will be very useful for young ophthalmologists worldwide.

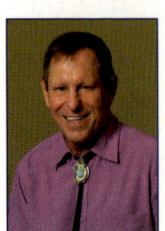

Professor Alan S Crandall
John A Moran Presidential Professor
Senior Vice-Chair of Ophthalmology and Visual Sciences
Director of Glaucoma and Cataract
Co-Director, Division of International Ophthalmology at the Moran Eye Center,
University of Utah in Salt Lake City, Utah, USA

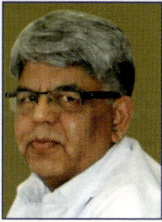

I am proud of our alumnus, Dr Suresh K Pandey, for bringing out this video atlas *State of Art in Ophthalmic Surgery*, which is in keeping with the changing times. Their videos are very thorough, and I particularly like the emphasis on Career Options and guidance for youngsters. I congratulate Dr Suresh Pandey and Dr Vidushi Sharma and I am sure this atlas will be of tremendous benefit to the ophthalmologists worldwide.

Professor Amod Gupta
Professor and Head
Department of Ophthalmology
Advanced Eye Center, PGIMER, Chandigarh, India

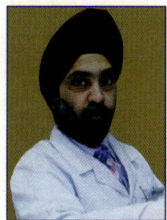

I am happy to see the video atlas *State of Art in Ophthalmic Surgery* compiled by Dr Vidushi and Dr Suresh Pandey. This series covering various ophthalmic surgeries is sure to be a big help for trainee students and practicing ophthalmologists alike.

Dr Mahipal S Sachdev
Director, Center for Sight Group of Eye Hospitals
New Delhi, India

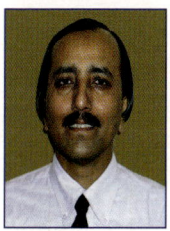

Congratulations to Dr Suresh Pandey and Dr Vidushi Sharma for bringing out video atlas *State of Art in Ophthalmic Surgery*. Watching surgical videos with explanation is one of the best teaching aids, and this video atlas covers most of the commonly performed anterior segment surgeries, particularly in phacoemulsification. This will be a very useful aid for all ophthalmologists who are interested to learn or master ophthalmic surgeries.

Professor Jagat Ram
Professor of Ophthalmology
Advance Eye Center, Post Graduate Institute of Medical Education and Research, Chandigarh, India

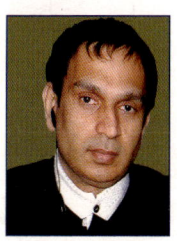

I congratulate Dr Suresh Pandey and Dr Vidushi for this video atlas *State of Art in Ophthalmic Surgery*. Section on phacoemulsification and premium IOLs is very comprehensive and discusses various aspects of phacoemulsification in different and difficult, challenging situations. Dr Suresh and Dr Vidushi have done a wonderful job with this atlas that will be very helpful for ophthalmologists worldwide.

Professor Amar Agarwal
Director
Dr Agarwal Group of Eye Hospitals, Chennai, India

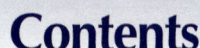

Contents

Section 1: Phacoemulsification Surgery

Section 2: Premium IOLs (Multifocal, Toric and Multifocal Toric)

Section 3: Piggyback IOL Implantation

Section 4: Pediatric Cataract Surgery

Section 5: Glaucoma Surgery

Section 6: Career Choices for Ophthalmologists Today

Section 7: Social Media and Medical Professionalism in the Changing World

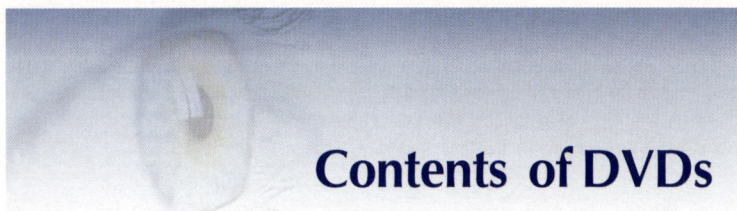

Contents of DVDs

1 Section

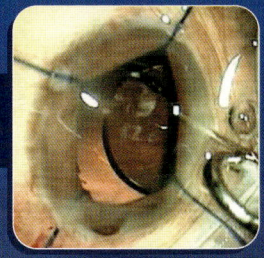

Phacoemulsification Surgery

1

Pearls for Phacoemulsification in Small Pupil

Vidushi Sharma, Suresh K Pandey

Eyes with small pupils present a challenge to cataract surgeons. A pupil that fails to dilate can obscure visualization during all stages of phacoemulsification, making surgery more difficult and increasing the incidence of complications such as nucleus drop, vitreous prolapse, and iris tear. Inadequate pupil dilation is often seen in patients with a history of use of miotic agents, chronic uveitis, diabetes mellitus, pseudoexfoliation syndrome, intraoperative floppy iris syndrome (IFIS), iris trauma, and rubeosis iridis.

Fortunately, the availability of several intraoperative techniques and pupil-expanding devices enables phaco-emulsification to be performed even in these difficult eyes. Strategies for enlargement primarily depend on the surgeon's skill level and preference and on the individual intraoperative situation. This article presents pearls for a variety of methods used to facilitate phacoemulsification in patients with small pupils.

Viscomydriasis

A highly cohesive ophthalmic viscosurgical device (OVD) such as Healon 5 (Abbott Medical Optics Inc.) can be used to manipulate a small pupil intraoperatively. As phaco-emulsification progresses and the OVD is washed out of the anterior chamber, the pupil will become small again, at which point reinjection of the OVD can help to redilate the pupil. In such cases, it is important to perform slow-motion phaco-emulsification and to maintain minimal turbulence so that the OVD stays within the anterior chamber and is not rapidly washed out. The bottle height must be low to achieve low fluidics and ensure that the OVD stays within the anterior chamber. Remember to remove all of the OVD at the end of the case, especially from under the IOL.

Malyugin Ring

Pupillary expansion devices such as the Malyugin Ring (MicroSurgical Technology) can also be used to enlarge a small pupil. The Malyugin ring is a square-shaped implant with four circular loops that hold the iris at equidistant points; it is available in two sizes, 6 and 7 mm, and conveniently comes with its own injector.

The Malyugin ring is injected through the main incision, and the four scrolls are placed on the iris to enlarge the pupil. Normally, the three scrolls that emerge first can be engaged fairly easily, and then a second instrument is needed to position all of the scrolls on the iris in an optimal manner. This device provides uniform dilation and protects the iris all around. Phacoemulsification can then proceed as in any normal case.

The main advantages of the Malyugin ring are that:

1. Its use does not require the creation of any additional incisions,
2. It is simple to inject,
3. It does not take long to deploy, and
4. It provides a uniformly dilated pupil and protects the iris. In all cases, it is again important to perform careful and gentle phacoemulsification to reduce the amount of stress placed on the zonules. Also, because the pupil can create problems at later stages in the case, we must be careful to perform slow-motion phacoemulsification and ensure that the procedure goes smoothly. Again, OVD should be used very generously in all of these cases; therefore, it is important to remove all of the OVD from the capsular bag, especially from under the IOL.

At the end of the case, the Malyugin ring is removed with the injector (Fig. 1.1). The scrolls must first be freed carefully from the iris margin. The iris sometimes becomes edematous during surgery, and, therefore, pulling on the scrolls without

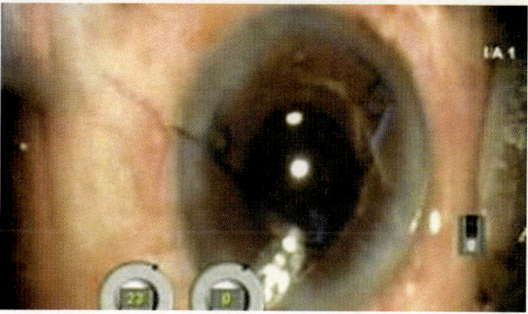

Fig. 1.1: *Malyugin ring*

freeing them initially has been reported to cause iridodialysis. Once all of the scrolls are freed, one of the scrolls is engaged in the Malyugin ring injector, and the ring is withdrawn through the same incision that was used for injection.

Iris Retractors

Iris retractors have been available for a long time and can be used to facilitate phacoemulsification in patients with small pupils. Four iris retractors are used in each case; therefore, the disadvantage of this approach is that four additional paracentesis incisions must be made. Most surgeons prefer to place the iris retractors in a diamond configuration (Fig. 1.2),

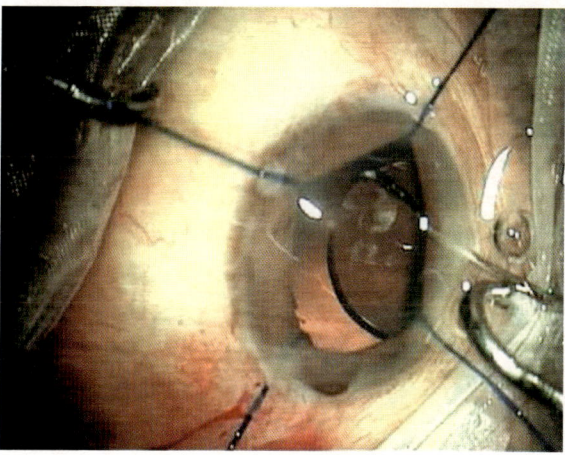

Fig. 1.2: *Iris retractors*

as this provides greater visualization inferiorly, where most phaco movements take place.

Iris retractors may tend to slip off as the case progresses, especially if the retractor is placed subincisionally. The surgeon should be careful not to rotate the globe too much, as that increases the chances of the iris retractors slipping out. If the retractors do slip out, they should be placed back in again, taking care not to catch the capsulorrhexis edge with the hook.

Pupil Stretch (Fig. 1.3)

In the case of a small pupil due to a thick fibrotic iris, a pupil-stretching technique using two Kuglen hooks can be employed. This technique is most suitable for postuveitic, thick fibrotic irides, which can be mechanically dilated with the use of iris hooks. However, it is important not to stretch the iris too much or apply too much sudden force, as this may cause the iris to tear. Therefore, the increase of force must be gradual. It is a good idea to slightly enlarge the pupil first with pupillary stretching and then use viscomydriasis to enlarge it further.

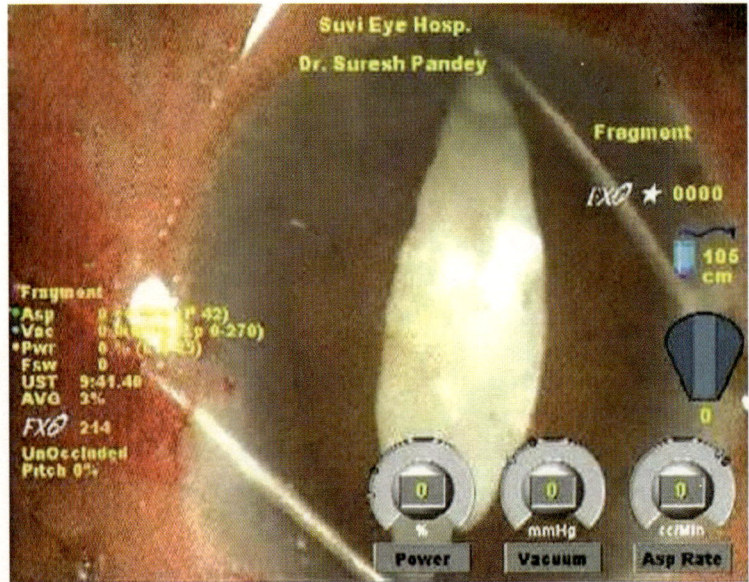

Fig. 1.3: *Pupil stretch*

It has been suggested that the pupillary stretching technique releases prostaglandins and causes increased inflammation, and that it should therefore be avoided. The technique does, however, have some role in selected eyes with postuveitic, fibrotic irides. One should also remember not to perform pupillary stretching in patients with IFIS, as this will make the iris even more floppy, causing it to prolapse out of the incision.

Intracameral Dilation

Intracameral injection of preservative-free lidocaine 1% can be used to achieve pupillary dilatation. This technique is not successful in all cases; however, if it does not work, intracameral lidocaine can be further supplemented with the use of viscomydriasis to achieve a fairly well dilated pupil, and capsulorrhexis and phacoemulsification can be performed as in any standard case.

The use of epi-Shugarcaine, a term coined by the late Joel K. Shugar, MD, has been described to help achieve pupillary dilation in patients with IFIS. This combination of buffered lidocaine and epinephrine provides intracameral anesthesia and also helps to overcome the action of alpha-1-blockers such as tamsulosin HCl (Flomax, Boehringer Ingelheim) that are often responsible for IFIS. This approach can also be used as a supplement to other techniques when the pupil is stubbornly small or constricts during phacoemulsification.

Conclusion

Pharmaceutical agents, intraoperative techniques, and surgical devices can all be used to facilitate phacoemulsification in patients with small pupils. Depending on surgical skill, preference, and scenario, a combination of these techniques and technologies can make it safe to perform phacoemulsification in these difficult eyes.

2

Phacoemulsification in Traumatic Cataract in Adult and Pediatric Cases

Suresh K Pandey

Trauma is a common cause of unilateral cataract. Prevention of eye injuries is of utmost importance and is the team responsibility of parents, teachers, coaches, ophthalmologists, pediatricians, and optometrists. Traumatic cataract can present many medical and surgical challenges to the ophthalmologist. Comprehensive examinations, careful planning for surgical management, and close follow-up are necessary for a favorable outcome in these cases. We suggest primary repair of the injury first and cataract IOL surgery after 2 to 4 weeks of topical steroid and atropine treatment. This delay may be helpful in achieving the optimum surgical outcome by reducing the postoperative inflammation in these eyes and allowing healing to occur. Long delays before cataract removal must be avoided during the amblyopia-prone years, which extend to approximate the age of 8 years.

Cataracts caused by blunt trauma classically form stellate— or rosette-shaped posterior axial opacities that may be stable or progressive, whereas penetrating trauma with disruption of the lens capsule forms cortical changes that may remain focal if small or may progress rapidly to total cortical opacification. Anterior and/or posterior capsule defect, intralenticular foreign body, partial/total zonular loss, dislocation, and subluxation of the lens are often found in combination with traumatic cataract. Other associated complications include glaucoma (phacolytic, phacomorphic, pupillary block, and angle recession), phacoanaphylactic uveitis, retinal detachment, choroidal rupture, hyphema, retrobulbar haemorrhage, traumatic optic neuropathy, and globe rupture. Anterior

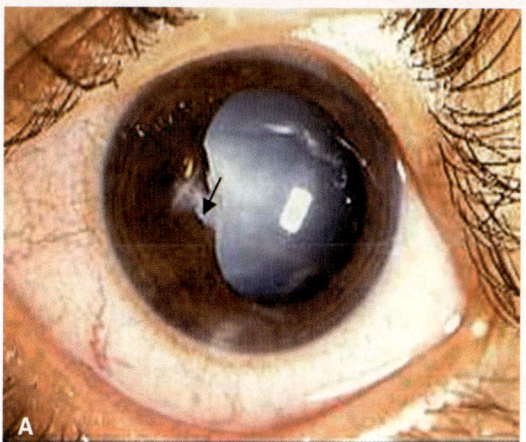

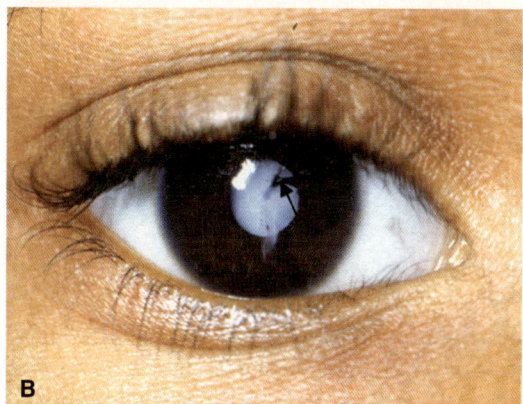

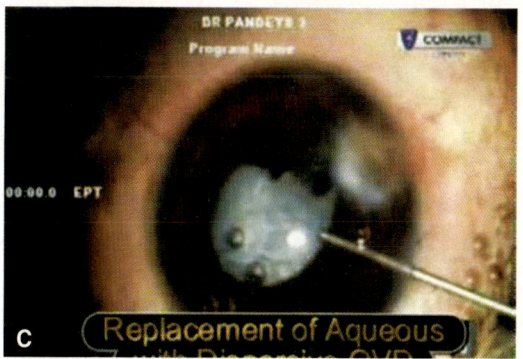

Fig. 2.1: *Traumatic cataract in children*

capsule rupture (with flocculent lens matter in the anterior chamber) may be associated with an increased IOP and/or possible lens-induced uveitis (e.g. phacoanaphylactic and phacotoxic endophthalmitis).

In the setting of traumatic cataract, the ophthalmologist must first examine other ocular injuries in detail. The cataract surgeon should be suspicious of injury to other ocular structures. Management depends on the degree and type of injury. Localized traumatic cataracts (especially if not in the visual axis) may be managed conservatively, while more significant lens opacities generally require cataract extraction. Similarly, capsular perforation may be managed with observation if small and not centrally located. Frequently, such injuries will develop only very localized opacification of the underlying cortex, without progression to generalized cataracts.

The initial patient evaluation is one of the most important critical steps in the management of any traumatic cataract. Data gathered during this examination, to a large extent, direct further investigations and establish immediate priorities. One of the most important aspects of this first examination is the description of the exact circumstances of the injury. This facilitates the development of risk estimates for occult injuries, such as IOFB, chemical exposure, and posterior rupture of the globe. A *guarded prognosis* for anatomical and functional outcome is to be thoroughly explained to the patient and the patient's relatives. The full extent of the eye injuries is not always known prior to cataract surgery. The patient and relative must understand that IOL implantation is not always possible at the initial surgery. It is also important to explain about the possible need for additional surgeries depending on the type of injury (retinal detachment, keratoplasty for dense corneal scar obstructing visual axis, etc.). The use of an IOL in traumatic cataracts is well accepted. It offers a constant, maintenance-free optical correction and, as such, helps in the prevention of amblyopia. Malplacement of the IOL is more common, in traumatic cataracts since damage to the capsular bag, zonules, and iris may predispose to decentration and pupil capture. In addition, contact lens wear may be helpful after ocular trauma to help compensate for an irregular corneal curvature caused by a healed corneal wound. However, children often have difficulty wearing these lenses due to discomfort and poor motivation to wear the lens.

TRAUMATIC CATARACT—TIMING OF SURGERY

The timing of traumatic cataract surgery in children is important. Some authors have reported IOL implantation at the time of primary repair. While the development of amblyopia in children necessitates prompt removal of a cataract when it develops, in our experience, cataract surgery is not necessarily required at the time of initial repair even when anterior capsular rupture is present. We prefer to defer cataract surgery and IOL implantation while the inflammatory response is treated with topical steroids. Cataract surgery with IOL implantation can often be safely delayed to allow a complete evaluation of damage to intraocular structures. It is important to rule out associated injury (e.g. posterior capsule rupture, vitreous hemorrhage, and retinal detachment) using ancillary methods such as B-scan ultrasonography and to allow healing after the primary repair. However, medically uncontrolled ocular hypertension may occasionally necessitate earlier cataract surgery. Cataract surgery and IOL implantation (combined during the primary repair of ocular trauma) may be considered in younger children predisposed to amblyopia.

Surgical Steps for Pediatric Traumatic Cataract Surgery

- *Anesthesia:* General anesthesia is preferable even in older children who might otherwise be cooperative for local anesthesia.
- *Incision:* Although corneal tunnel incisions have become routine, we recommend a scleral tunnel incision when operating on a traumatic cataract. The integrity of the capsular bag and the zonular support is often in question. If conversion from a planned foldable IOL insertion to a rigid PMMA IOL insertion is needed, scleral wounds are more easily enlarged to the 6- to 7-mm length that may be required.
- *Synechiolysis:* Traumatic cataracts are often associated with posterior synechiae and it is necessary to perform synechiolysis in these eyes. Iris repositor instruments or high-viscosity viscoelastic material can be used for this purpose.

- *Anterior capsule management:* Management of the lens capsule in traumatic cataract cases may be difficult due to a ruptured lens capsule with flocculent lens matter in the anterior chamber. Creation of an intact capsulorhexis may be difficult in such a situation. Staining of the anterior lens capsule may be helpful to enhance visibility in these eyes with a "torn anterior capsule" or "white cataract." Anterior capsule staining can be successfully done using a nontoxic capsular dye such as 0.1% trypan blue (Fig. 2.2).

Anterior Capsule Staining in Pediatric Traumatic Cataract

- *Hydrodissection:* Avoid doing *hydrodissection* in such cases if the integrity of the posterior capsule is suspicious.
- *Posterior capsule and vitreous management:* Management of the posterior capsule depends on the age of the patient and status of the posterior capsule (intact versus torn). In young patients (too young to sit still at the Nd:YAG laser) with complex trauma, proper placement of the IOL is paramount. If this can be accomplished best by leaving the posterior capsule intact at the initial cataract surgery, plan a

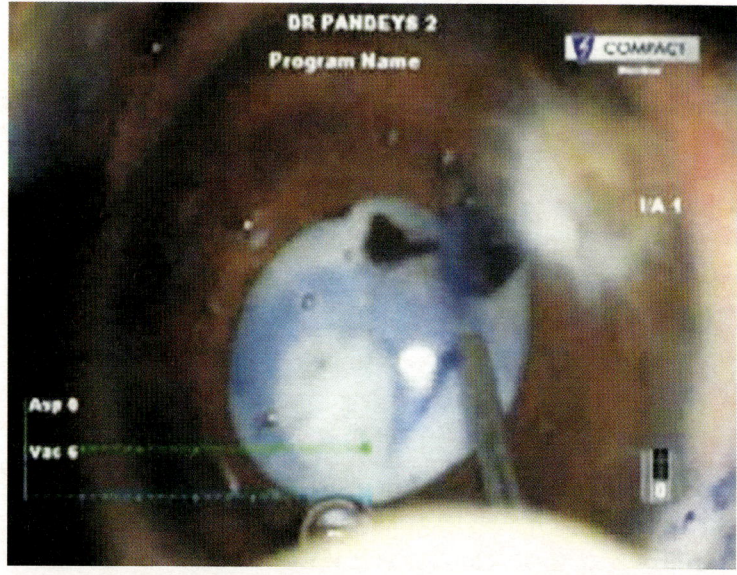

Fig. 2.2: *Anterior capsule staining in pediatric traumatic cataract*

secondary surgery to remove the center of the posterior capsule after the IOL has become healed into the lens capsule. This staged approach may be better for surgeons unaccustomed to operating on young children. PCO occurs quickly in most cases of complex traumatic cataract surgery. Therefore, prepare the family that the best vision will likely come after this planned second surgery. Repair of iris defects or other more elective surgical maneuvers can also be done during this secondary procedure, which is often done 4 to 8 weeks after the initial cataract removal.

- *IOL implantation*: Continued advances in IOL designs, biomaterial, and power calculations are making this decision easier in the pediatric population. In-the-bag placement of the IOL haptics improves implant stability and minimizes uveitis and pupillary capture. In-the-bag fixation is believed by most to be the best site for IOL implantation, as it sequesters the implant from uveal structures, reduces the chance of lens decentration, and delays PCO formation. However, traumatic cataract cases often present unique challenges, as it is not always possible to fixate the IOL haptics in the capsular bag due to anterior and/or posterior capsule tears from trauma or the difficult surgical procedure. If the IOL must be placed in the ciliary sulcus, as with extensive traumatic posterior capsule rupture, try to capture the IOL optic through the anterior capsulotomy. If this can be done, it will eliminate the risk of pupil capture. Since the iris sphincter is often damaged in trauma, pupil capture of sulcus-fixated IOLs is higher in traumatic as opposed to nontraumatic IOL sulcus fixation.

- *Removal of corneal suture:* Do not forget to remove corneal sutures from the original traumatic globe rupture repair if they are present and wound healing has been completed.

- *Postoperative medication:* Depending on the case, we may sometime increase the frequency of steroid drops. Also, a short course of systemic steroids may be indicated. If IOP control had been a problem after the original trauma, perhaps during hyphema resolution, it is likely that elevated IOP will be seen transiently after cataract surgery. Prophylactic oral Diamox is recommended during the early healing phase in such cases.

Complications

The main postoperative complications following pediatric cataract surgery with IOL implantation include PCO and/or secondary membrane formation, pupillary capture, IOL precipitates, and decentration/dislocation of the implant. We continue to recommend planned primary posterior capsulotomy in children too young to undergo an awake Nd:YAG laser capsulotomy. Occurrence of pupillary capture can be reduced after precise fixation of the IOL within the capsular bag. The one eye that developed pupillary capture after in-the-bag IOL placement had a ruptured anterior capsule and iris damage prior to IOL implantation. Had it been possible to maintain an anterior capsular opening smaller than the IOL optic, pupillary capture could have been avoided. Iris-to-posterior capsule adhesions re-formed in this patient, causing recurrence of the pupillary capture. Decentration/dislocation of an IOL can occur because of traumatic zonular loss and/or inadequate capsular support. Capsular bag placement of the IOL combined with a capsule tension ring is a reported method that may be helpful in the presence of zonular dehiscence/loss. Capsular Tension Segments (CTS) are recommended when the integrity of the posterior capsule has been breeched. Posterior capture of the IOL optic may be useful, at times, to obtain better centration of the implanted IOL. Asymmetric IOL fixation, with one of the haptics in the capsular bag and the other in the ciliary sulcus, can also lead to decentration and should, therefore, be avoided. Complete IOL dislocation can occur after trauma. Explantation or repositioning of the IOL may be necessary in some cases presenting with significant decentration/dislocation.

3

Phacoemulsification of the White Cataract

Vidushi Sharma

Phacoemulsification of white cataracts is associated with some difficulties and a higher rate of intraoperative complications. Like any fear, the fear of the white cataract can be overcome through preparation and repeated exposure. The use of vital dyes for staining the anterior capsule enhances visualization and helps perform continuous curvilinear capsulorrhexis, which is a key point for performing successful phacoemulsification.

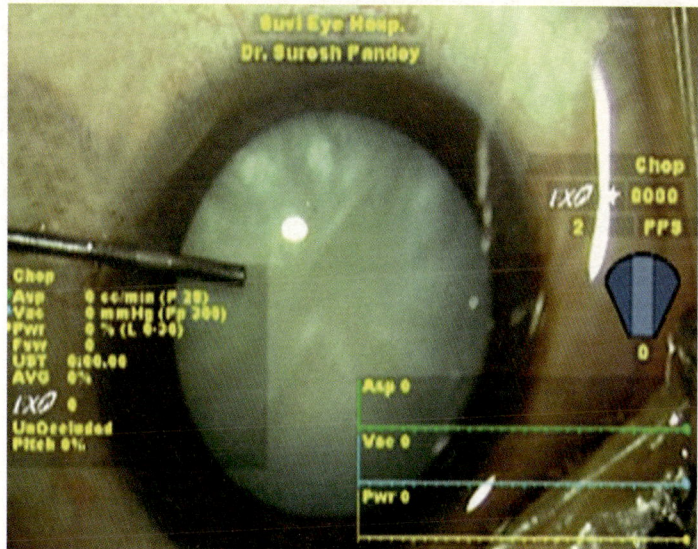

Fig. 3.1

Challenges of White Cataract

Operating on a white cataract requires that you must be prepared to deal with the following challenges:

- The absence of a red reflex
- A pressurized capsular bag
- A liquid cortex
- An unpredictable anterior capsule
- A dense nucleus with large mass
- The absence of an epinucleus.

By addressing each of these features, phacoemulsification can proceed smoothly in these difficult cases.

The Absence of a Red Reflex

The absence of a red reflex in a white cataract is the first challenge that must be addressed. Capsular dyes such as trypan blue allow us to subdue this monster fairly easily. We combat the absence of a red reflex by using capsular dyes, allowing us to visualize the edge of the capsulorhexis as it progresses. Phacoemulsification is made possible through the

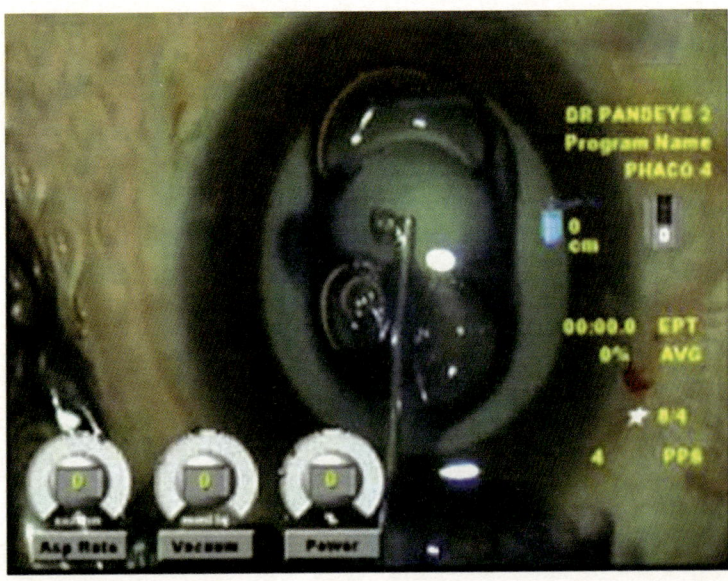

Fig. 3.2

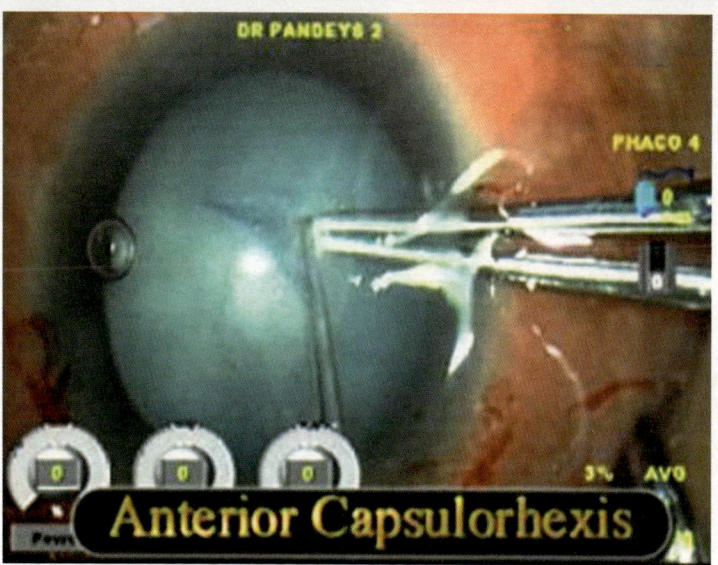

DR PANDEYS 2

PHACO 4

3%   AVO

Anterior Capsulorhexis

Fig. 3.3

presence of an intact capsulorhexis. Without a red reflex, capsulorhexis is exceedingly difficult.

After placing the paracentesis and intracameral lidocaine, trypan blue is introduced into the anterior chamber. The simplest method is to inject the dye directly into the aqueous, without the placement of an air bubble. This can adequately stain the capsule. However, because the trypan blue will be diluted by the volume of the aqueous, the stain is not as intense as when the trypan blue is injected under an air bubble. If you prefer a more intense stain, then inject the dye under an air bubble, directly onto the anterior capsule. Rather than injecting air via a separate syringe, it is simpler to inject the air and the dye with the same syringe. After drawing up approximately 0.2 cc of trypan blue into a TB syringe and placing a 26-gauge cannula on the syringe, hold the syringe with the tip down and draw up 0.1 cc of air. The air will stay in the proximal part of the syringe (nearest to the cannula), allowing you to inject both the air and trypan blue with a single entry of the cannula into the anterior chamber. Next, inject viscoelastic into the anterior chamber, replacing the trypan blue and/or air bubble. The anterior capsule is now visible for capsulorhexis despite the absence of a red reflex. Perform your phaco incision as usual. We have shown some videos without using trypan blue but this should not be tried by the beginner.

A Pressurized Capsular Bag

In many cases of white cataracts, the cortex has liquefied and the capsular bag has positive internal pressure. With a normal cataract, the initial puncture of the anterior capsule by the cystotome is a rather ordinary event. However, with a white cataract, puncturing the pressurized capsular bag can lead to extension of the capsular incision across the entire capsule, resulting in a gash of exposed lens across the center, from one side of the iris to the other, with a swath of capsule on either side of the gash. The striped appearance of capsule-lens-capsule resembles the flag of Argentina—known as "Argentinian Flag" sign during surgery. The edges of the anterior capsulotomy are ragged and extend across the entire anterior capsule, disappearing behind the iris. In fact, it is difficult to be sure whether or not the capsular gash has extended beyond the equator onto the posterior capsule. An Argentinian Flag makes the rest of the phaco extremely challenging because there is no intact capsulorhexis and many times the extent of the capsular tear is unknown. In order to avoid this explosive extension of the initial capsular puncture, overfill the anterior chamber slightly with viscoelastic. This additional pressure in the anterior chamber helps tamponade the capsule and minimize the risk of explosive extension of the initial capsulorhexis incision.

A Liquid Cortex

Not all cases of white cataract have liquefied cortex, but many do. With the placement of the initial capsular puncture, the liquid cortex can rapidly leak out of the bag and obscure the view of the capsule through the liquid cortex mixed with viscoelastic in the anterior chamber. At this point, one solution is to introduce the irrigation/aspiration (I/A) tip, remove the liquid cortex and viscoelastic from the anterior chamber and reinflate the anterior chamber with new viscoelastic before proceeding with the capsulorhexis. However, because at this point the capsulorhexis is far from complete, there is risk of extension of the anterior capsular tear by introducing irrigation and positive pressure into the anterior chamber. If you do choose to remove the liquid cortex with I/A, I strongly recommend using a manual technique with the Simcoe I/A where the irrigation and the aspiration can be delicately controlled and performed slowly.

We have found the following option simpler in dealing with the liquid cortex. In making the initial puncture for the capsulorhexis, use a 25-gauge needle as a cystotome. With a single motion, puncture the anterior capsule and enter the anterior cortex of the lens. Begin aspirating the liquid cortex immediately. Some cortex will likely leak into the anterior chamber. However, with aspiration of the remaining liquid cortex while it is still in the capsular bag, leakage into the anterior chamber can be minimized and visibility of the anterior capsule will be maximized.

A White Cataract Taunts the Surgeon through a Mid-dilated Pupil

The small amount of liquid cortex that leaks into the anterior chamber can be aspirated by moving the cystotome tip anterior

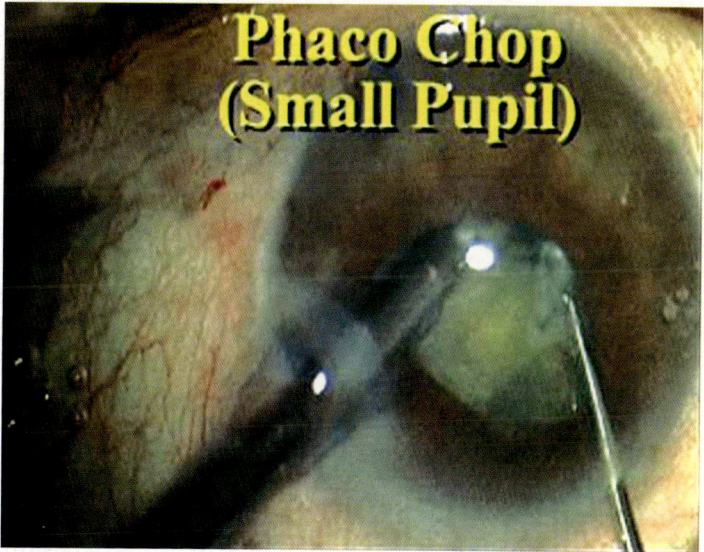

Fig. 3.4

to the anterior capsule and into the anterior chamber. However, the more cortex that is aspirated while it is still in the bag, the easier it will be. Once it mixes with the viscoelastic, it becomes more difficult to aspirate. The puncture and aspiration is a delicate move. If the puncture is too deep or the aspiration too vigorous, your cystotome can go through the posterior capsule. That's not good. So be decisive, quick and gentle in puncturing the anterior capsule and aspirating the liquid cortex from the bag.

The capsulorhexis can then be continued. Sometimes, liquid cortex remains sequestered in parts of the bag and may be encountered during the progression of the capsulorhexis. In most cases, these small amount of liquid cortex do not interfere with visualization. If they do, they can be displaced by the addition of more viscoelastic, which also serves to deepen the chamber.

An Unpredictable Anterior Capsule

As you begin the capsulorhexis, you may notice that the capsule is not behaving as usual. It may be either very elastic and difficult to tear, or it may be friable and rip easily. Some surgeons advocate making a large capsulorhexis when performing phaco on a white lens; however, we have found that a small capsulorhexis is best. By keeping the capsulorhexis small, it is easier to prevent straying of the capsulorhexis to the periphery. This is particularly important in light of the unpredictable nature of the anterior capsule. A large rhexis is more likely to extend peripherally, and with the unusual capsular elasticity with a white cataract, it is very difficult to recover. The smaller capsulorhexis also serves to contain the waiting segments of the nucleus in the posterior chamber during phacoemulsification, helping to keep these large chunks from drifting anteriorly and touching the corneal endothelium.

The Large Dense Nucleus

In some white lens cases, the nucleus may be very soft and can be removed in the usual phaco-chop technique with typical ultrasound powers. Impaling the nucleus with the phaco tip can serve as a test of its density. If it is not unusually hard, you

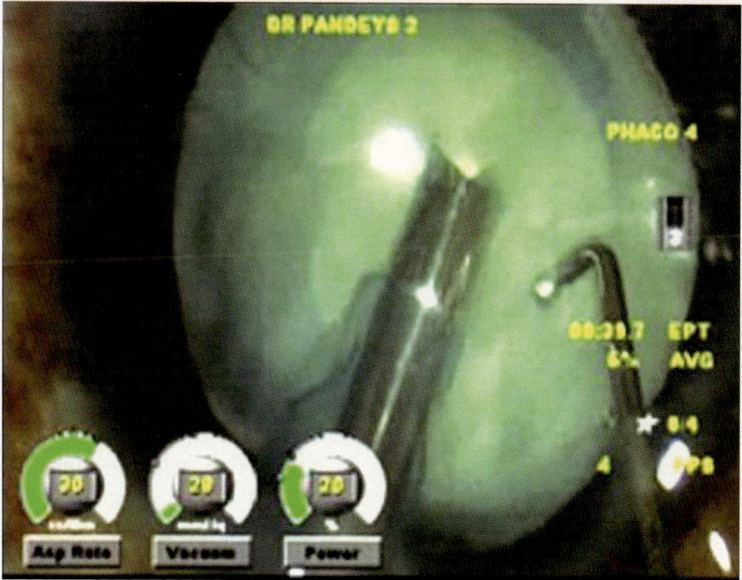

Fig. 3.5

may use your regular chopper and begin the horizontal phaco chop process. However, if the nucleus is too dense for a horizontal phaco chop, as is often the case, you need to prepare for vertical chopping.

As a first step in the battle against the size and density monster, excavate a central bowl in the nucleus to about 2/3 to 3/4 nuclear depth. This process serves three purposes. First, it debulks the nucleus. The mass of the nucleus can be huge. Removing a significant portion of the nucleus while it is held stable within the capsular bag eliminates the risk of damaging the corneal endothelium or posterior capsule if you try to remove that same mass later when the pieces are mobile and the posterior capsule exposed. Second, the bowl creates space for the subsequent removal of the first segment of the nucleus. And third, by thinning the central nucleus, it makes propagation of the vertical chop through the posterior central plate of the nucleus easier.

Excavation of the bowl usually goes smoother by moving the silicone sleeve of the phaco tip back, exposing more of the phaco tip. If the sleeve is close to the tip, it can interfere with excavation, getting hung up on the sides of the bowl as you get deeper. Also, while excavating the bowl, the tip can often get stuck in the distal dense nucleus. This can be prevented by removing the proximal portion of the nucleus—that portion closest to the phaco incision—rather than the distal nucleus. Rotate the nucleus frequently to maximize the symmetry of the central excavation, which helps ensure even segments in subsequent chopping.

After the central bowl is excavated, vertical chopping may begin. The phaco tip is driven into the distal side of the bowl at about 2/3 depth, obtaining a firm grasp on the nucleus with the phaco tip. The sharp chopper is then used to come down vertically through the nucleus toward the impaled phaco tip. The vertical chop is performed centrally. The sharp chopper should not be placed beneath the edge of the anterior capsule, as it may stray to the periphery and inadvertently puncture the posterior capsule. As a right-handed surgeon, I usually chop down toward the center of the phaco tip. Once I near the tip, I pull the chopper horizontally toward the left and the phaco tip toward the right. This lateral movement helps to separate the segments, and to propagate the chop. Many times, a white nucleus can be leathery and it can be difficult to separate the segments, but this lateral movement can help significantly.

Depending on the size of the nucleus, it may require segmenting the nucleus into six or eight portions. Complete all the chops before removing any of the segments. This helps ensure that the volume of the bag remains stable, keeping the posterior capsule protected while the sharp chopper is in the eye.

A central bowl and vertical chopping have slain the fifth monster. Now, switch to your usual chopper and begin removal of the nuclear segments.

The Absence of an Epinucleus

Because the nucleus can be so large and dense, or the cortex liquefied, there is often very little epinuclear material to protect the posterior capsule. As the first segment of nucleus is removed, you will now have a bare, unprotected posterior capsule visible and exposed while removing the remaining

80% or so of the nucleus. A few techniques can help protect the posterior capsule.

We recommend phacoemulsifying centrally and relatively anteriorly, just below the anterior capsular plane, in the anterior third of the posterior chamber. Using phaco power in the periphery or more posteriorly is more likely to lead to posterior capsular tears. Performing the phacoemulsification in the anterior chamber or iris plane puts the corneal endothelium at risk, especially in light of the higher phaco times needed to remove the large nuclear mass.

Use viscoelastic generously during the phacoemulsification to form a cushion between the nuclear fragments and the posterior capsule—a sort of "viscoelastic epinucleus." Viscoelastic should also be used throughout the case to protect the corneal endothelium, especially in light of the longer phaco times. You may also turn the blunt chopper upside-down and use the broad knuckle of the chopper to keep the posterior capsule back away from the phaco tip.

While removal of white nuclear fragments requires that you visualize the phaco tip at all times. Emulsification of each segment must be deliberate, and requires patience.

Finally, paradoxically, the case becomes riskier as more of the nucleus is removed, because it leaves more of the posterior capsule bare, unprotected by cortex or epinucleus, and exposed to the phaco tip. In cases where the posterior capsule is particularly floppy and unpredictable, as in previously vitrectomized eyes, we use viscoelastic to displace the final small nuclear segment into the anterior chamber. I will then insert the posterior chamber IOL beneath the nuclear fragments. The IOL serves to stabilize and protect the posterior capsule. I then complete removal of this final nuclear segment with phacoemulsification in the anterior chamber. With the posterior chamber lens in place, the posterior capsule is protected. (The final fragments can also be removed by viscoexpression.)

Phacoemulsification in White Cataract without Preoperative Dilating Eye Drops

Intracameral injection of preservative-free lidocaine (0.2 cc of Oculan) was attempted as an alternative to reduce the potential

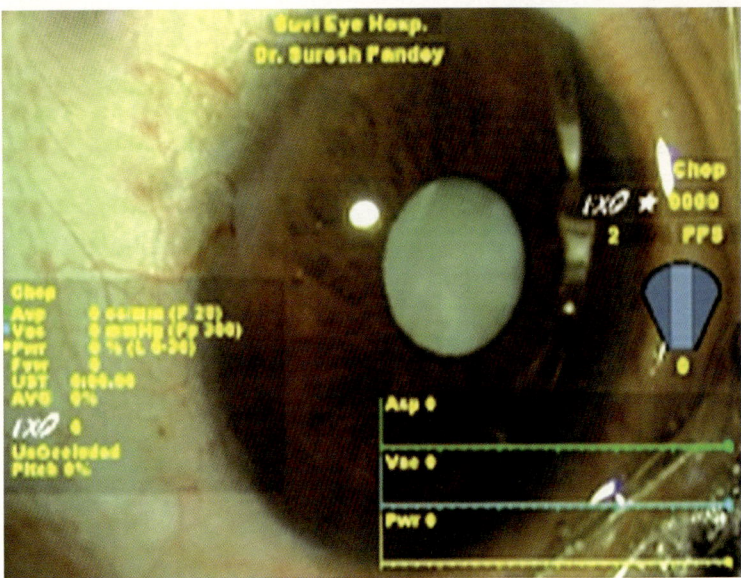

Fig. 3.6: *Before injection of intracameral lignocaine*

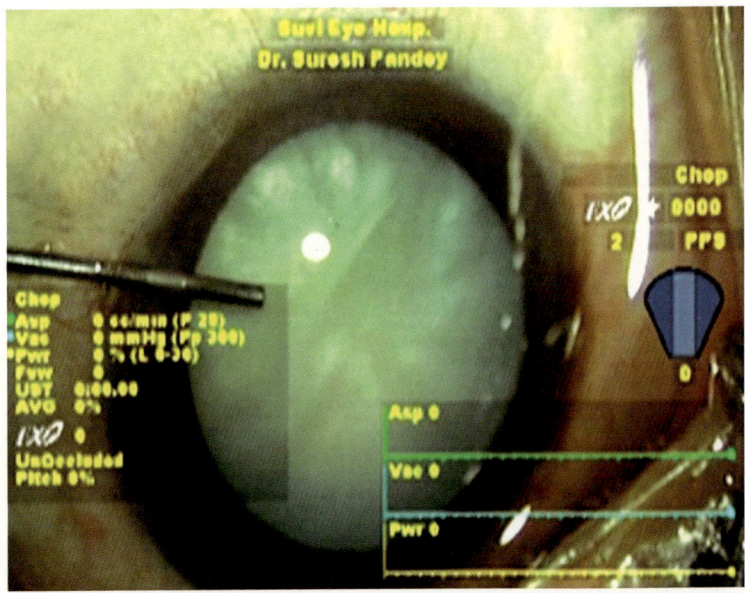

Fig. 3.7: *After injection of intracameral lignocaine (Notice pupil dilatation)*

disadvantages of common mydriatic eye drop. Intracameral lidocaine has some advantages over topical mydriatics. It does not need time-consuming preoperative program for pupillary dilation, does not have systemic side-effects of topical mydriatics and provides satisfactory pupillary dilation as well as simultaneous anesthetic effect in phacoemulsification cataract surgery.

4

Phacoemulsification in Postural Disorders

Vidushi Sharma, Suresh K Pandey

Phacoemulsification is routinely performed with the patient lying supine with his or her head flat to optimize the red reflex and surgical view. If a patient has a medical condition that precludes lying supine, then both the patient and surgeon may be uncomfortable. If the surgeon's view is compromised due to poor positioning, the potential risk for complications increases.

Positioning can be challenging in a variety of medical conditions, including kyphosis, chronic obstructive pulmonary disease, congestive heart failure, cerebral palsy, myotonic dystrophy, obesity, and Ménière disease. With simple modifications to the patient's position, successful, uncomplicated cataract surgery can be performed.

CASE REPORT

A 56-year-old man presented with a decrease in vision due to age-related cataracts in both eyes. He had severe congenital kyphosis and was unable to lie flat on the operating table (Fig. 4.1). The patient consulted other ophthalmologists, but most were uncomfortable performing cataract surgery because he was unable to lie flat.

We performed a mock drill in the operating room to determine the best position for the procedure, which involved adjusting the microscope and phaco machine footpedal. The patient was seated on the operating table with the help of a few pillows (Fig. 4.2).

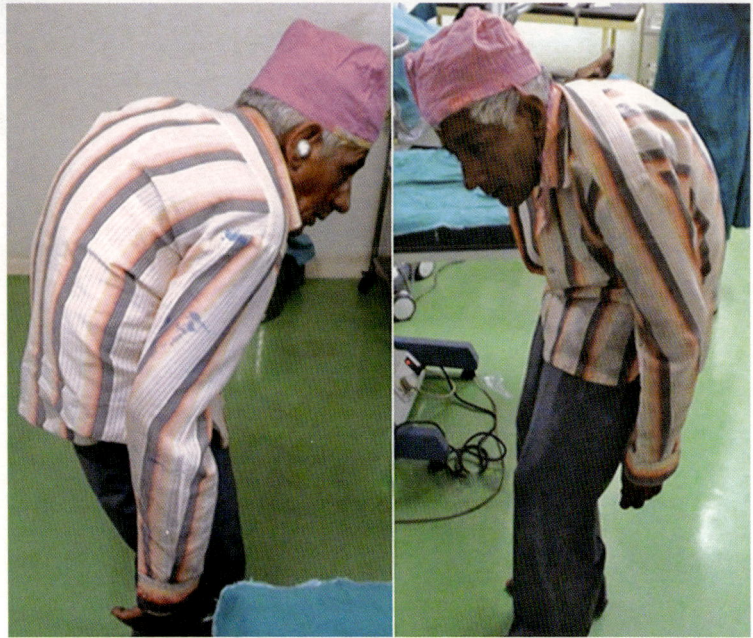

Fig. 4.1

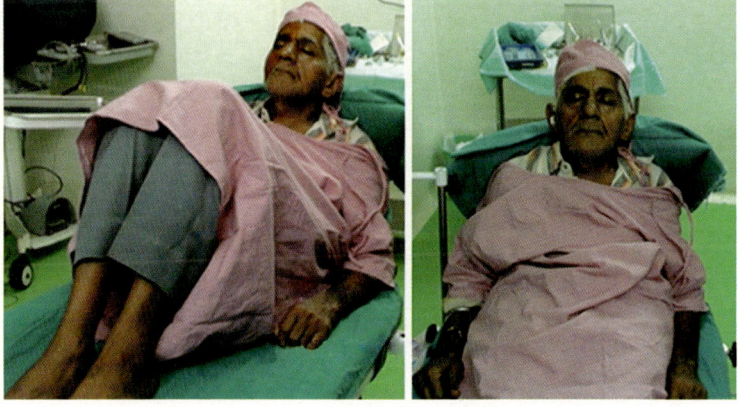

Fig. 4.2

With the patient seated and the surgeon standing (Fig. 4.3), standard phacoemulsification under topical anestheisa with the white star signature system with the ellips transverse ultrasound handpiece (Abbott Medical Optics Inc.) was performed in the patient's right eye, and a Sensar foldable IOL (Abbott Medical Optics Inc.) was implanted in the capsular

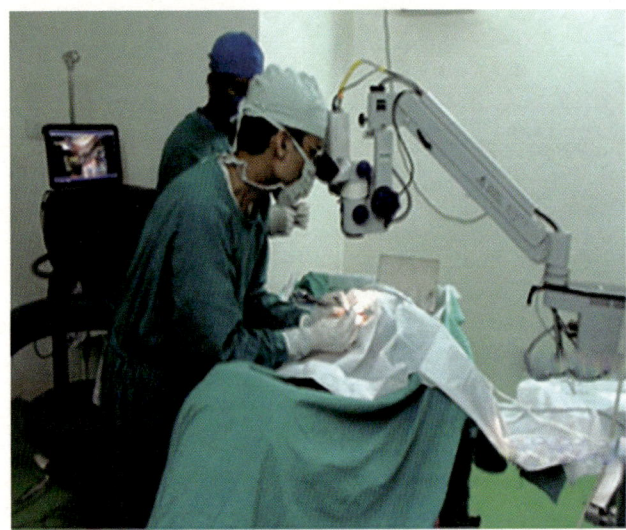

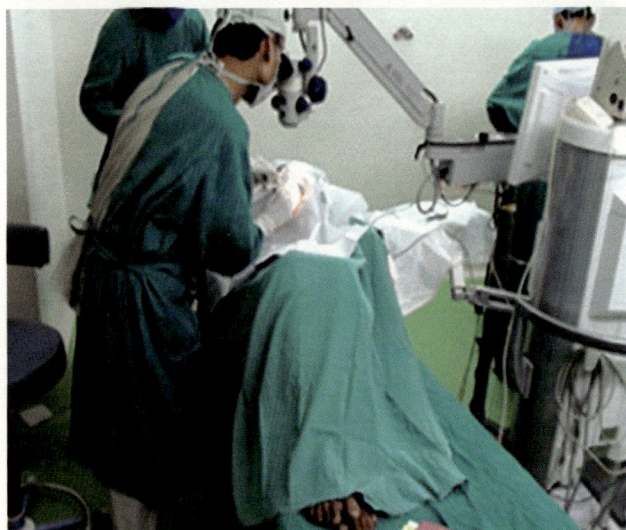

Fig. 4.3: *Surgeon performing phacoemulsification in standing posture*

bag. The surgical procedure was uneventful; postoperatively, the patient achieved 20/20 UCVA in his right eye.

Techniques for Postural Disorders

No. 1: Face-to-face position: Ang et al positioned a patient seated in a standard reclining cataract surgical chair in an almost upright position. They rotated the ceiling-mounted surgical microscope 60° from the vertical to point toward the patient. The surgeon sat beside the patient, and, while facing him or her, operated at nearly arm's length. Topical anesthesia without sedation was used, which, according to the authors, allowed the patient to follow requests regarding where to fixate. With the surgeon's arms outstretched and at an unfamiliar angle, an inferior surgical approach via a clear corneal incision at 270° was used. Ang and colleagues reported using this face-to-face positioning technique for two patients, neither of whom experienced intra- or postoperative complications. To date, it has not been reported in the literature that an inferior approach would lead to greater postoperative complications compared with normal positioning.

No. 2: Standing phacoemulsification in reverse-Trendelenburg position: Mansour et al described a standing phacoemulsification technique for morbidly obese patients. For this technique, the surgeon was standing, the surgical microscope was at minimum magnification and in the maximum upward position, and the patient was in reverse-Trendelenburg position. This position may help lower posterior venous pressure by reducing central venous pressure. Patients with morbid obesity face a variety of health complications including increased risks of cataracts and elevated intraocular pressure.

No. 3: Side-saddle position: The side-saddle position is an alternative to standing when using the operating microscope. The patient is positioned on the operating table at the lowest inclination tolerable, and the operating microscope's axis is tilted back 60° toward the horizontal. The footpedals are placed parallel to the long axis of the operating table. The patient's head is rotated toward the surgeon and/or in a chin-up position. The surgeon sits side-saddle with his or her thighs parallel to the long axis of the operating table and facing the head of the bed. The globe is tilted slightly more superotemporal than usual to optimize visualization of the red reflex, and an inferotemporal surgical approach is used.

This approach is familiar to surgeons who operate from the side of the table. Surgery performed in this position may be facilitated with topical anesthesia, allowing the patient to fixate according to the surgeon's request. The more upright the patient is, the more the operating microscope must be adjusted toward the horizontal. Consequently, the surgeon's arms will be more outstretched. The surgeon must decide whether he or she is more comfortable sitting side-saddle or standing.

No. 4: Phacoemulsification in a standard waiting room chair: Modifications can be made to a standard waiting room chair for patients with both respiratory disease and claustrophobia. Fine et al altered a common waiting room chair, attaching an adjustable headrest to the back of it, thus allowing the patient to remain seated upright with his or her head tilted back but supported. Other minor adjustments were made to the chair, such as adding weights for stability and lowering the height so that a patient's legs extended outward to provide counter-balance. This technique is useful for patients who can tolerate sitting with their head extended back.

Conclusion

Orthopedic, neurologic, cardiovascular, and pulmonary conditions can affect patients' positioning during cataract surgery. Adjusting the operating chair and/or table, rotating the surgical microscope, altering the surgical approach, and using pillows are effective techniques for managing patients unable to lie supine during the procedure.

5

Phacoemulsification in Black/Rock Hard Cataract

Vidushi Sharma

Phacoemulsification of the extremely dense cataract poses challenges for even the most experienced cataract surgeon. The absence of a protective epinuclear layer, the paucity of cortex, the fragility of the capsule, and the laxity of the zonules all increase the risk of injury to the supportive structures of the lens during surgery. Longer phaco times at higher energy levels, moreover, increase not only the risk of corneal endothelial damage but also the risks of mechanical or thermal injury to the iris or cornea. Successful surgical management of these cases requires planning and careful attention to detail.

Anterior capsulorhexis (CCC) remains crucial step for managing black cataract and surgeons should aim for a relatively larger CCC. Trypan blue provides a more intense and persistent coloration, which enhances visibility of the capsulorhexis edge during emulsification.

The surgeon should perform multiquadrant hydrodisscetion and be careful to avoid capsular block during hydrodissection. To avoid capsular-lenticular block, one should terminate hydrodissection as soon as the solid nucleus elevates against the capsulorhexis. One must avoid the temptation to continue injecting until the migrating posterior fluid wave completely crosses behind the nucleus. Instead, tap the center of the elevated nucleus to dislodge it posteriorly before resuming hydrodissection from the opposite quadrant.

PHACO IN BLACK CATARACT

Burst mode and high vacuum combine to provide a maximal grip. Inadequate holding power makes it more likely that the

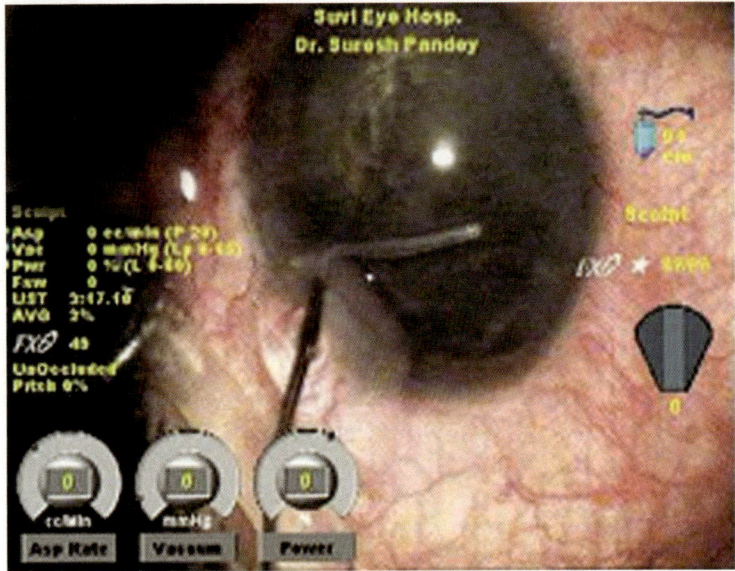

Fig. 5.1

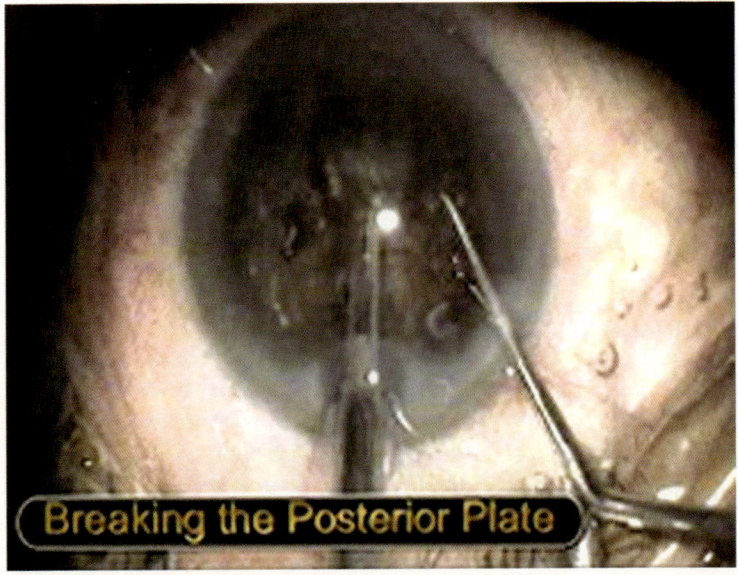

Fig. 5.2

vertical chopper will dislodge pieces from the phaco tip, and makes it more difficult to elevate large fragments out of the bag. Particularly with a brunescent lens, continuous mode cavitation cores out the firm material surrounding the phaco tip. This facilitates sculpting but prevents total tip occlusion by eroding the seal. Because high vacuum levels require a well-occluded phaco tip, burst mode is particularly advantageous for the dense lens. It is important to sculpt a central pit prior to diagonal phaco chop. By reducing phaco power and time as well as stress on the zonules, chopping is a superior phaco technique for the brunescent nucleus. In the absence of an epinuclear shell, horizontal phaco chop is contraindicated, and vertical chop also is better able to transect the leathery posterior plate. Sculpting a deep pit in the central anterior nucleus allows the surgeon to penetrate the bulky nucleus more deeply and peripherally with the phaco tip than if the nucleus was impaled without this step. To better impale the nucleus, one should maximally retract the irrigation sleeve and bury the tip to the hilt. A very sharp vertical chopper will best incise into the dense nuclear face without displacing it. We like to first place the chopper peripherally beneath the blue-stained anterior capsule, and then chop in a diagonal direction toward the buried phaco tip. This adds a slight horizontal vector force that compresses the fragment against the phaco tip during the vertical chop. The surgeon can subchop brunescent fragments in to create smaller "bite size" fragments. Regardless of whether the initial nuclear fragmentation is accomplished by divide-and-conquer, stop-and-chop or pure chopping methods, the resulting fragments are much larger and denser than those encountered with typical nuclei. One can employ horizontal chopping to subdivide these large fragments into smaller, bite-sized pieces. This reduces the tendency for oversized fragments to deflect away from the vibrating phaco tip. By reducing particle chatter and turbulence within the anterior chamber, endothelial cell loss can be lessened. Hyperpulse power modulation is now available from a number of phaco machines. The widely recognized advantages of hyperpulse are a dramatic reduction in heat and energy production, and improved followability because of decreased chatter of fragments at the phaco tip. The combination of subchopping and hyperpulse mode can significantly reduce particle turbulence within the anterior chamber, which we believe is the most important factor in decreasing endothelial cell loss with brunescent cataracts. With the prolonged operative times associated with brunescent nuclei, viscoelastic washout is a far greater problem than with most typical cases. Dispersive viscoelastics, such as Viscoat, or the viscoadaptive Healon 5, if utilized properly, are able to coat and protect the endothelium for longer periods than their cohesive counterparts. As all viscoelastics eventually wash away, consider stopping to replenish the protective endothelial layer midway through the nuclear removal step.

Even when proceeding with phaco, the surgeon must have a contingency plan for unexpected problems such as weak zonules or poor visibility. For the most challenging cases, consider administering a regional anesthetic block—and have a contingency kit of instruments needed to convert to a standard ECCE/SICS readily available.

6

Phacoemulsification in Soft Cataract

Vidushi Sharma, Suresh K Pandey

Plenty of videos are available demonstrating phaco techniques for hard cataracts; but, in many ways the soft cataracts are the most challenging. Soft cataracts tend to jump to the phaco needle which can lead to capsule rupture. Soft cataracts are hard to crack which can make the divide and conquer very difficult. With soft cataracts, the inexperienced surgeon may unexpectedly sculpt through the nucleus too rapidly, as well as aspirate and possibly phaco the posterior capsule. In this video we demonstre a few strategies for soft cataracts to increase safety for these tricky lenses.

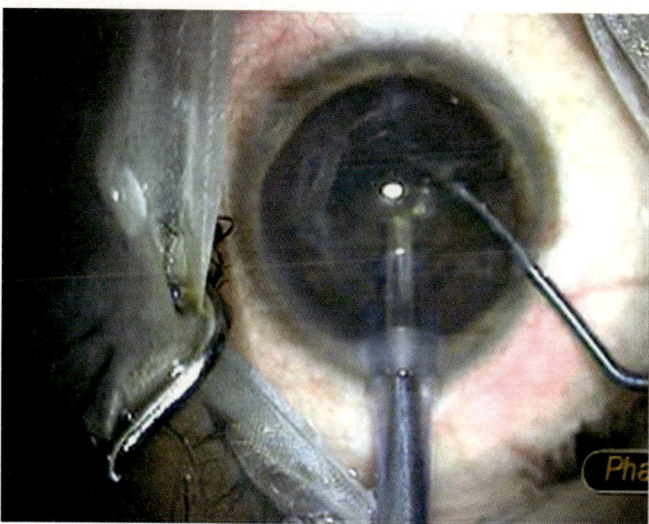

Fig. 6.1

The simplest strategy for very soft cataracts is to simply prolapse the soft lens into the iris plane/anterior chamber. Even better is to prolapse just the nucleus. First we like to hydrodissect, careful to keep the cannula over the lens, to avoid prolapse. Then spin the lens. Then perform hydro-delineation and allow the nucleus to prolapse into the iris plane/anterior chamber. In a perfect world you can just prolapse the nucleus (sometimes soft lenses have a denser central core) and leave the epinuclear material in the bag. Then remove the nucleus with the phaco needle with epinuclear settings (linear control of vacuum 0–350, asp at like 30–35 fixed, little power). Remove the epinuclear material with the phaco needle and a shizzle maneuver or with the I/A tip. The technique I like best for the soft cataract is to use a soft chop with no vacuum. Avoiding vacuum is very important as the phaco needle can rapidly move through the soft lens material into the capsule. The idea is to use the phaco needle to hold and support the soft lens while slicing through the lens with the chopper.

7

Phacoemulsification in Posterior Polar Cataract

Vidushi Sharma

A posterior polar cataract presents a special challenge to the phaco surgeon because of its predisposition to posterior capsular dehiscence during surgery. A posterior polar cataract is a dense white opacity that is situated on the central posterior capsule. Posterior polar cataract is a congenital condition that can be sporadic or familial. Sporadic posterior polar cataracts are typically unilateral and associated with remnants of the tunica vasculosa lentis, an embryologic hyaloid structure that

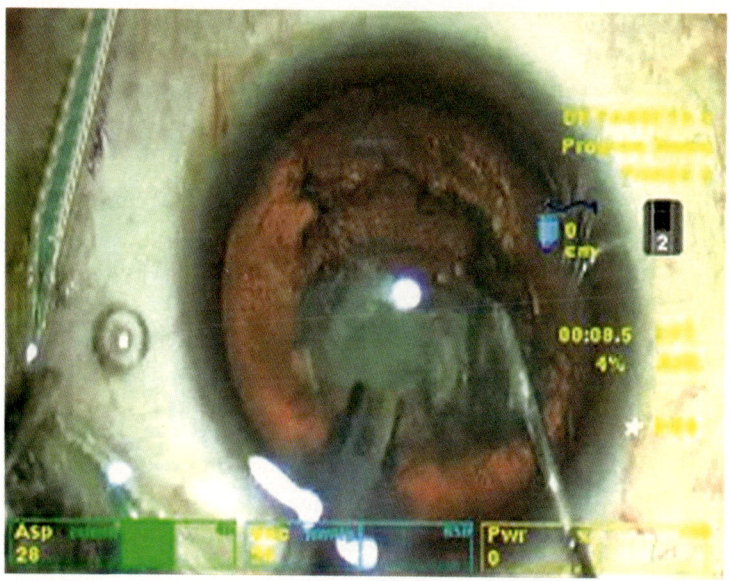

Fig. 7.1

fails to regress. Familial posterior polar cataracts are typically bilateral and follow an autosomal dominant pattern of inheritance. More recently, mutations resulting in a 17-base-pair duplication in the PITX 3 gene have been associated with posterior polar cataract. This gene codes for a transcription factor that participates in anterior segment and lens development. The exact mechanism of how the mutation causes cataract is unknown, but the result is dysplastic, abnormal lens fibers that, as they migrate posteriorly from the equator, form an opacity in the region of the central posterior capsule. The opacity is usually a round discoid plaque, clearly demarcated from the rest of the lens and often associated with vacuoles in the lens surrounding the plaque. Satellite opacities, which may represent fluid entering the lens, can also develop with time around the original plaque. The abnormal lens fibers can become adherent to the central posterior capsule, and the capsule around the plaque is often weakened. Thus, posterior capsular rupture is a feared complication when removing this type of cataract. These cataracts often present in the first few months of life, and if visually significant at an early age, can lead to amblyopia. Most posterior polar cataracts are stationary but can progress in severity over time.

How to Perform Safe Phaco in Posterior Polar Cataract?

When posterior polar cataracts become visually significant (either in infancy if the cataracts are large enough to be amblyogenic, or in adulthood when they cause glare), they can be surgically removed. However, the high risk of posterior capsular rupture makes surgical removal often very difficult. There have been reported rates of posterior capsular rupture in 26–36% of cases depending on the series studied. More recent studies demonstrate lower rates of posterior capsular rupture. To avoid posterior capsular rupture the following techniques have been described in the literature.

- *Injection of viscoelastic:* Avoid injecting excessive viscoelastic into the anterior chamber as the increased anterior pressure can cause posterior capsular rupture.
- *Capsulorhexis:* Avoid a large anterior capsulotomy. In the setting of a posterior capsular rupture, a large opening may not provide enough support for a sulcus intraocular lens.

- **Hydrodissection:** Avoid hydrodissection as the fluid wave can cause rupture of the weak posterior capsule. Visco-dissection can be safely utilized if the nucleus has been debulked as was demonstrated in the above video.
- **Hydrodelineation:** "Inside-out delineation" is a technique described by Dr Abhay Vasavada. A central bowl or trench is made in the anterior epinuclear material using low phacoemulsification settings as proposed by Dr Rober H Osher. The low vacuum level and aspiration flow rate provide a more stable anterior chamber and reduce the risk of surge, which can cause chamber collapse, anterior posterior movement of the iris lens diaphragm, and strain on the zonules and capsule. Low bottle height prevents the posterior capsule from ballooning. After this initial sculpting, the nuclear material is hydrodelineated from the epinuclear material by carefully placing the tip of the syringe in the central lens material and slowly injecting fluid in this plane until a golden ring is seen. This "inside-out" hydrodelineation technique can avoid the inadvertant injection of fluid in the subcapsular plane, which can lead to posterior capsular rupture.
- **Lens rotation:** This step should be avoided.
- **Nucleofractis:** Aspirate the nuclear material if the nucleus is soft, or use slow motion phacoemulsification (example: bottle height 60 cm, vacuum 100–150 mm Hg, and aspiration flow rate at 20 ml per minute) to gently remove nuclear fragments within the epinuclear shell, which was created by hydrodelineation.

8

Phacoemulsification in a Patient of Radial Keratotomy

Vidushi Sharma

Eyes that have undergone radial keratotomy (RK) present two separate challenges to the refractive cataract surgeon. First, the altered and often irregular curvature of the cornea after RK renders standard keratometry and routine IOL calculations inaccurate. Second, the altered anatomy of the post-RK cornea with its compromised structural integrity leads to technical challenges during phaco surgery. Linear RK incisions were typically made in a spoke-like pattern extending from a 3–4 mm central optical zone peripherally to within 1–2 mm of the limbus. The incisions were made to 90–95% corneal stromal depth and numbered from 2 up to 32 or higher in some extreme cases. Most spherical myopic RK treatments involved 4–16 radial incisions arranged in a symmetric wagon wheel spoke pattern over the cornea. Various incisions for the treatment of astigmatism were often added as T-cuts or other small concentrically arranged incisions placed between and perpendicular to the radial cuts. At the time that RK was in widespread use, cataract surgery was still mainly performed via scleral incisions either in the form of extracapsular cataract extraction or scleral tunnel phaco surgery. Consequently, there was little worry at the time about how these peripherally located corneal RK incisions would interfere with future clear corneal cataract surgery. Unfortunately, we now find ourselves dealing with this unintended legacy as we take care of an increasing number of post-RK presbyopic hyperopes and cataract patients.

Challenges of phaco in RK patients: Inaccurate IOL calculations, extended postoperative recovery and patients' mindset create the possibility of a difficult procedure. Because of their irregular corneas, even mild cataracts can induce visually significant aberrations at an earlier stage than would be expected for a traditional patient. This is a difficult subset of patients for many reasons: The IOL implant calculations can be inaccurate, the surgical procedure can be challenging, and the postoperative recovery can be prolonged. However, the greatest challenge is often the mindset of the refractive patient. These patients often have high demands and are frequently intolerant of residual refractive errors.

Pearls for IOL Power and Type Selection

Many formulas and techniques have been described for calculating IOL power in post-radial keratotomy (RK) patients. This tells me that there is no single method that yields great results. The principal error in calculation is overestimation of the corneal power, which results in implantation of a lower power IOL and postoperative hyperopia. Because these patients have typically been myopic their entire lives, leaving them with residual hyperopia is particularly uncomfortable and bothersome. To help prevent postoperative hyperopia, a more myopic result can be targeted, such as -0.75 D instead of the typical -0.25 D.

In patients with no old records, the method that we use most often to calculate corneal power was proposed by Robert K. Maloney, MD. It uses the central corneal power as measured by topography, and therefore, does not depend on history. The power of the cornea is a combination of the anterior corneal power and the posterior corneal power. By converting the overall central corneal power from topography back to the anterior corneal power, then subtracting the expected posterior corneal power, we can achieve a fairly accurate estimation for our IOL calculations. This formula is:

Estimated K power = (Central K power on topography $\times$ 376/337.5) $-$ 6.1.

Because of the irregular corneas, we prefer to avoid multifocal IOLs, instead preferring single focus lens implants. Aspheric IOLs may be a particularly good choice in these patients because of their significant corneal aberrations.

Implanting a negative spherical aberration aspheric IOL can help to offset the large amount of positive spherical aberration often seen in RK corneas. In this case, we prefer the advanced medical optics TECNIS IOL, as it has the best ability to offset large degrees of corneal positive spherical aberration. When the corneal aberrations are not known and a degree of irregularity and other higher order aberrations are suspected, we prefer the Bausch & Lomb SofPort Advanced Optics, as it has zero spherical aberration and is the "do no harm" IOL that will not confound the aberrations.

Surgical Pearls for Phacoemulsification

In patients with previous 8-cut RK, clear corneal incisions can be made between the existing RK incisions. In patients with 16-cut or more RK, it becomes difficult to avoid the existing RK incisions unless a scleral tunnel cataract incision is used (Fig. 8.1).

To be gentle on the weakened cornea, we prefer lower flow and a lower bottle height with a smaller phaco needle to ensure

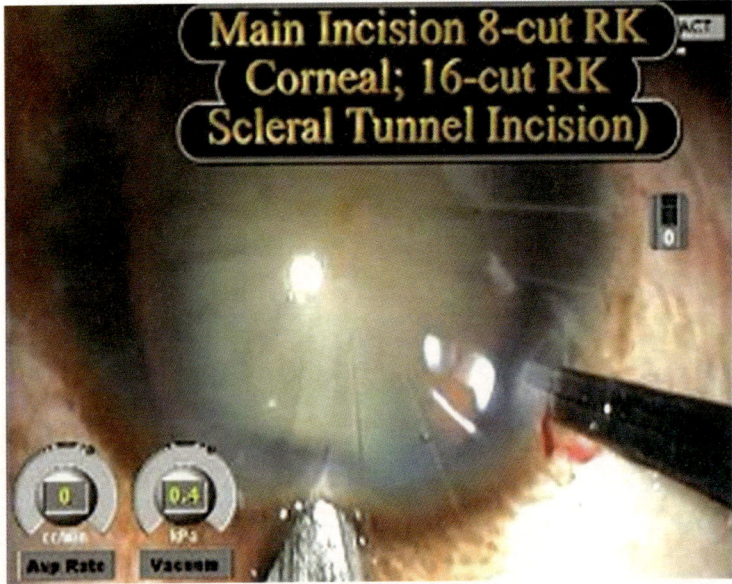

Fig. 8.1: *The RK incisions are weak and are prone to opening during surgery. Any incisions made during cataract surgery must avoid intersecting the existing RK incisions, lest they unzip and cause excessive fluid leakage during surgery*

that the fluid inflow still stays greater than the fluid outflow. If the RK incisions open during surgery, be aware that there could be sudden instability and shallowing of the anterior segment, and the chance for capsule rupture is increased. At the end of these surgeries, we like to paint the entire cornea with fluorescein dye to check for any leaks, which can easily be sutured while the patient is in the operating room.

Postoperative visual outcome: The RK incisions swell during even the gentlest cataract surgery, and this swelling can induce central corneal flattening, which results in excessive hyperopia immediately postoperative. These RK patients will experience fluctuations in their refractive state for many weeks after their cataract surgery, so a mild amount of initial hyperopia should not be a cause of concern. After waiting at least 6 weeks, if the patient is still significantly hyperopic, a second procedure can be performed. Perhaps the most important issues in RK patients with cataracts are explaining to them that their IOL calculations are, at best, estimations and that their surgery and postoperative recovery will likely be more challenging for the surgeon and the patient.

9

Phacoemulsification in Sub-luxated Cataract (Compromised Zonules)

Vidushi Sharma, Suresh K Pandey

In recent years devices and techniques were developed to preserve the capsular bag and maintain the capsular diaphragm between the anterior and posterior segments of the eye. Small zonular defects (up to 3 clock hours) can be treated using a capsular tension ring (CTR), however large defects require suture fixation of the capsular bag to the scleral wall. Modified endocapsular rings were developed, such as Cionni's ring (modified capsular tension ring—MCTR), Malyugin-Cionni ring and Ahmed's segment (capsular tension segment—CTS) (both manufactured by Morcher GmbH, Stuttgart, Germany). The modified rings support the entire (MCTR) or a part (CTS) of the capsular equator and are sutured to the scleral wall through an extension of the ring passing through the anterior capsulorhexis. *We discuss intraoperative clinical findings and strategies for managing compromised zonules during the early steps of cataract surgery, including capsulorhexis and hydrodissection, explaining the application of capsular tension rings and capsule retractors, devices that are especially helpful in weak zonule cases.*

Pearls for anterior capsulorhexis: The lack of zonular circumferential traction due to diffuse zonular weakness will create difficulty incising the anterior capsule, as though the cystotome were dull. If the cystotome tip depresses rather than incises the central anterior capsule, a halo-shaped light reflex may be noted. Finally, there may be significant phacodonesis as the cystotome first perforates and tears the anterior capsule. Weak zonules significantly increase the risk of a radial anterior capsular tear because of this pseudoelasticity. Because the

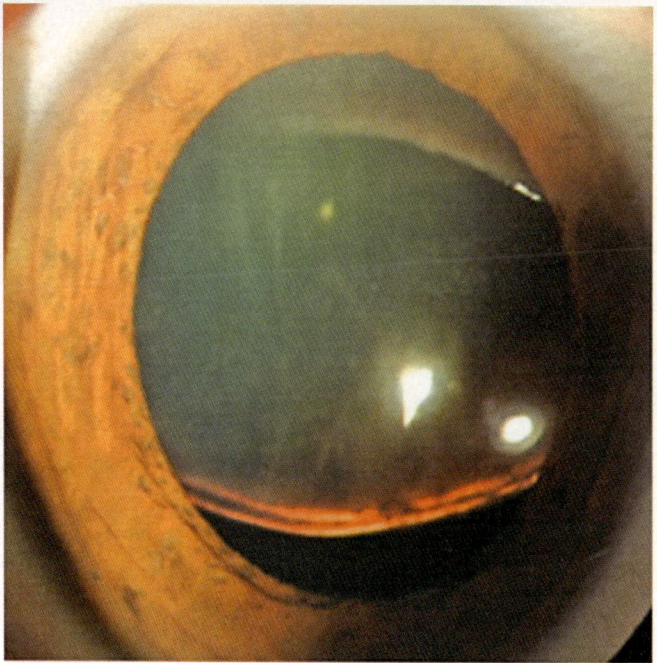

Fig. 9.1: *Sub-luxated cataract*

zonules do not adequately immobilize the anterior capsule, the peripheral capsule moves along with the flap as it is being torn. While a large diameter capsulorhexis would be helpful for phaco, making a smaller opening reduces the risk of a peripheral extension if one is struggling to control the tear.

Capsular retractors or a capsular tension ring (CTR) require a continuous curvilinear capsulotomy, the overriding importance of achieving an intact capsulorhexis dictates erring on the side of a smaller diameter that can be secondarily enlarged after the IOL has been implanted. The capsule tear-out rescue technique may be helpful for controlling a tear that wants to run radially because of weak zonules and pseudo-elasticity.

Pearls for hydrodissection: When there is diffuse zonular laxity, the nucleus is more difficult to rotate because of deficient capsular rotational stability and counter-fixation. One should therefore suspect significant circumferential zonular weakness if, despite proper and gentle hydrodissection technique (Fig. 9.2), the nucleus does not rotate easily. Overly forceful efforts to rotate the nucleus may shear already weakened zonules. This may potentially create a large zonular dialysis or dislocate the crystalline lens even prior to insertion of the phaco tip.

One alternative is to use two instruments to bimanually rotate the nucleus. In this situation, the second instrument tip, rather than the capsular bag, becomes the counter fixating fulcrum around which to rotate the nucleus. However, when severe zonular laxity is diagnosed during the capsulotomy step and the nucleus cannot be easily rotated following hydrodissection, the safest strategy is to insert capsule retractors. By fixating the capsular bag to the eye wall, capsule retractors will facilitate nuclear rotation and avoid creation of a zonular dialysis in the process.

Pearls for capsular tension rings (CTRs): There are some signals that must be cautiously evaluated during the slit lamp preoperative examination. While frank sub-luxation of the crystalline lens or extensive zonular dehiscence are easily evidenced, other aspects such as subtle iridodonesis or

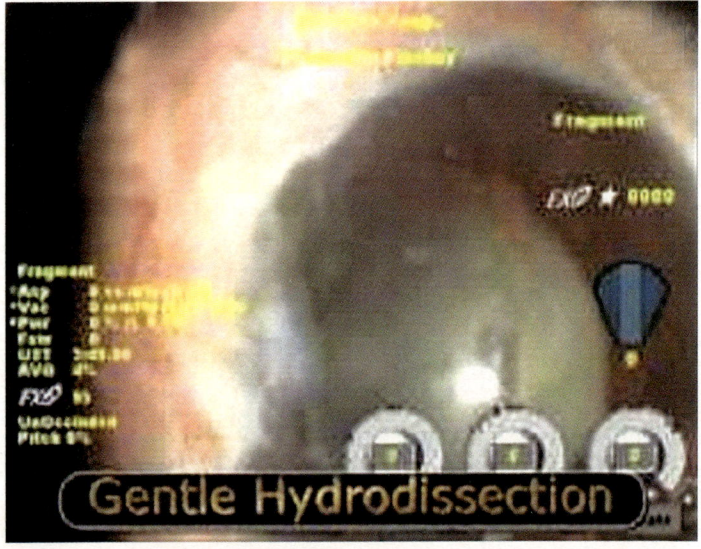

Fig. 9.2: *Gentle hydrodissection*

phacodonesis, deep anterior chamber, vitreous in the anterior chamber, increased retro-iridal space, and the presence of pseudo-exfoliative material at the papillary rim can be overlooked. These signals are frequently found in the following diseases: previous ocular trauma, Marfan's syndrome, high myopia, and previous intraocular surgery. These are situations where the implantation of capsular rings may be advisable (Fig. 9.3).

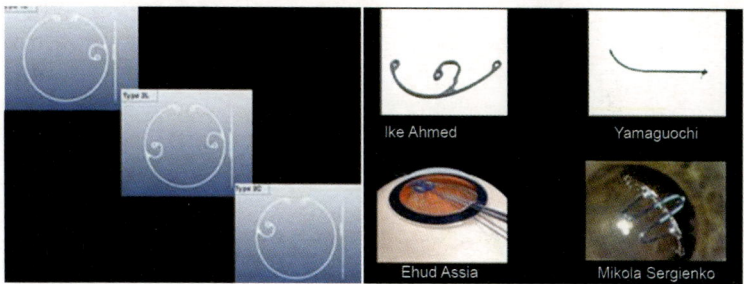

Fig. 9.3

In cases of mild zonular dialysis with little or no decentration of the crystalline, CTRs are enough to provide adequate stabilization of the capsular bag. They maintain the equator of the capsular bag fully distended in 360°, ensuing better conditions for the phacoemulsification and for the centration of the intraocular lens in the bag. The choice of the diameter of the CTR — in correlation to the size of the eye globe and or its dioptic power is not very important, as the implantation of a ring with a diameter bigger than that of the equator of the bag will only have the consequence of the overlapping of the extremities of the ring. On the other hand, choosing one with a diameter smaller than the diameter of the capsular bag will leave part of the capsular equator floppy.

The Cionni ring (CR) is the option when the dialysis is bigger than four clock hours and the sub-luxation of the crystalline is easily noticed through the well-dilated pupil. In the severe cases, one may choose the CR with two fixating eyelets instead of the model with one eyelet. As these eyes require additional delicate maneuvers at the ciliary body level and the surgery is lengthier than usual, topical anesthesia is not a good choice. In cases where a posterior capsular rupture is evidenced, both the CTR and the CR should not be implanted, as well as in cases of posterior polar cataract due to the higher risk of defective posterior capsule.

CTRs have two important disadvantages. Significant compression is required to implant the ring into the capsular bag because of its larger size. This may stretch the capsulorhexis and potentially shear zonules by ovalizing or decentering the bag. Because of this compressive rebound force, CTRs should never be inserted in the presence of an anterior or posterior capsule tear. Secondly, the ring may impede cortical aspiration by pinning and trapping cortex in the capsular fornix. Surgeons can delay CTR insertion by instead using capsule retractors to stabilize the bag during phaco. The capsule retractors should be left in place during CTR insertion to reduce zonular trauma.

CTRs compensate for weakened zonules in several ways. With a focal zonular weakness or dehiscence, the ring redistributes mechanical forces (e.g. from nuclear sculpting or IOL insertion) to areas of stronger zonular support. However, if the entire circumference of zonules is uniformly weak, this benefit is lost. A second advantage is that centrifugal pressure applied by the ring makes the flaccid capsular bag tauter. This reduces redundant capsule folds, forward trampolining of the posterior capsule, and inward collapsing of the capsular fornices toward the aspirating instrument tip. The final benefit of a CTR is to counter progressive contractile capsular forces postoperatively. Severe capsulophimosis is always a result of deficient zonular counter-traction and is a likely factor in spontaneous late dislocation of the entire capsular bag in pseudoexfoliation.

Pearls for Using Capsular Anchor

Ehud Assia, MD has developed "Capsular Anchor" an alternative device to fixate the intact lens capsule to the scleral wall (Fig. 9.4). The capsular anchor (Hanita lenses, Kibbutz Hanita, Israel) is a polymethyl methacrylate (PMMA) intra-ocular, uni-planer implant, inserted into the capsular bag after capsulorhexis is performed. The anchor clips, the anterior capsule, and supports a localized segment of the lens equator.

The two lateral arms of the device are inserted behind the anterior lens capsule, whereas the central rod is placed in front of the capsule. A 10–0, or preferably 9–0, prolene suture is used to fixate the anchor to the scleral wall. After lens removal by phacoemulsification a conventional PC-IOL is inserted into the capsular bag. The capsular anchor recently gained the CE mark and permit for use in Europe and is in use in several countries.

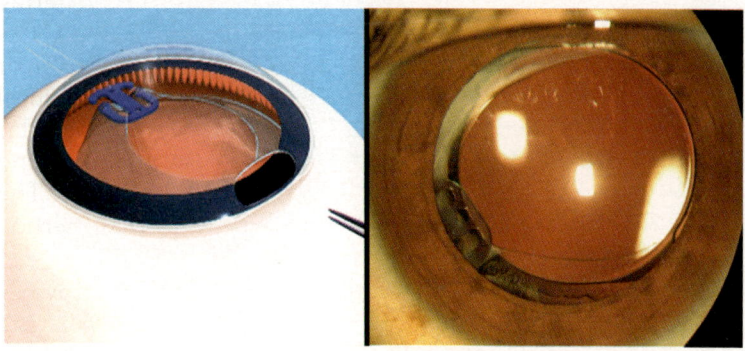

Fig. 9.4: *The capsular anchor. The 2 lateral arms are located behind the anterior capsule. The anterior central rod is placed in front of the capsule*

Pearls for inserting capsule retractors: In addition to enlarging a small pupil, flexible iris retractors can be used to support the capsular bag in the presence of extremely loose zonules. However, because the hooked ends are very short and flexible, iris retractors may tend to slip off of the anterior capsular edge during phaco and will not support the equator of the capsular bag. Richard Mackool, MD, designed capsular hooks that are elongated enough to support the peripheral capsular fornix and not just the capsulorhexis edge. In this way, the retractors function as artificial zonules to stabilize the entire bag during phaco and cortical clean-up. Unlike capsular tension rings, capsule retractors provide much better support in the anterior–posterior direction and do not trap the cortex. The disposable nylon capsular retractors from MicroSurgical Technology (Redmond, WA, USA) are a newer alternative to the Mackool Capsule Support System. Packaged three to a container, the former feature a double-barreled design that creates a loop at the tip, which is less likely to puncture the equatorial capsule.

Capsule retractors can be inserted through limbal stab incisions at any stage including midway through the capsulorhexis step. By anchoring the bag to the eye wall, the additional anteroposterior support and rotational stability facilitate hydrodissection and nuclear rotation. The self-retaining capsule retractors are also strong enough to center and immobilize a capsular bag that is partially sub-luxated due to a severe zonular dialysis. Finally, they restrain the peripheral anterior and equatorial capsule from being aspirated and dehisced by the phaco or I/A tip. As a single strategy for severe zonular deficiency, capsule retractors are significantly more effective than capsular tension rings at preventing posterior capsule rupture. Because CTRs can only redistribute instrument and mechanical forces to the remaining intact zonules, the greater the zonular defect or deficiency, the less effective a CTR is at stabilizing the bag. However, a CTR can be used in conjunction with capsule retractors, particularly if there is a sizable zonular dialysis. If after first inserting retractors the unsupported equatorial regions of the capsular bag tend to collapse inward toward the phaco tip, a CTR can be inserted to distend the equator of the bag to its proper anatomic configuration.

Although the tip of the capsule retractor is dull, it is possible for the hooks to tear the capsulorhexis margin during surgery. There is a tendency to over tighten the capsular retractors because the tension is initially adjusted with a soft eye. Inserting the phaco tip with irrigation suddenly displaces the nucleus and capsular bag posteriorly, which effectively further tightens the retractors. After inserting the phaco tip, it is therefore important to momentarily assess whether the capsule retractors have become so taut that they tent the capsulorhexis edge. If so, they should be loosened slightly so that the capsular rim does not tear during phacoemulsification. This is particularly important if the capsulorhexis diameter is on the small side.

Pearls for nuclear emulsification in compromised zonules: Fragile zonules are very prone to further damage during nuclear emulsification, and poor capsular bag stability heightens the risk of capsular rupture. Forceful sculpting or rotation of the nucleus may shear zonules in the oppositely located quadrants. Care should be taken to avoid causing excessive nuclear movement with sculpting, chopping, or rotation. Phaco chop significantly reduces the stress placed on the zonules and capsule by replacing sculpting and cracking motions with the manual forces of one instrument pushing inward against another. Because of the centrally directed instrument forces, horizontal chopping is particularly effective at avoiding nuclear tilt or displacement, and it is this author's preference for weak zonule cases. The supracapsular flip technique prolapses and flips the endonucleus out of the capsular bag prior to emulsification. If accomplished, this prevents the capsular bag from bearing any of the phaco instrumentation forces. The ease with which this flipping maneuver can be accomplished varies depending upon the size of the endonucleus relative to the capsulorhexis diameter. Using this technique with a nucleus that is too large or a capsulorhexis that is too small risks further zonular dehiscence. Care must also be taken to avoid endothelial trauma during the nuclear flipping maneuver. With chopping, one should consider bringing larger sections of nucleus out of the capsular bag where they can be sub-chopped within the supracapsular space. For example, it may be possible to lift each heminucleus out of the capsular bag following the initial bisecting horizontal or vertical chop.

Throughout phaco and cortical cleanup, one should anticipate that deficient centrifugal zonular tension will result in greater posterior capsule laxity. The flaccid posterior capsule will tend to trampoline toward any aspirating tip as the last nuclear fragments, epinucleus, and cortex are removed. Because the nuclear bulk will initially mask this situation, one must be vigilant as increasingly more nucleus is removed. Compared to a standard 19-gauge phaco tip, a smaller-diameter, 20-gauge tip greatly reduces the risk of inadvertently aspirating the peripheral or posterior capsule. If one suspects or encounters zonular laxity, the aspiration settings can be lowered as progressively more of the nucleus is removed. To slow the pace down, a lower than usual aspiration flow rate is advisable. A pre-programmed vacuum setting that usually avoids post-occlusion surge with routine cases may not be safe with a lax posterior capsule that is lacking normal centrifugal zonular tension. Therefore, one should consider decreasing the vacuum to lower than normal levels to prevent trampolining of the capsule. Repeatedly inflating the capsular bag with a dispersive OVD (Alcon Viscoat) can further restrain a flaccid posterior capsule from vaulting toward the aspirating instrument as the final fragments and epinucleus are aspirated. This is especially important if there is no epinuclear shell remaining as the last nuclear fragment is emulsified. Finally, placing the chopper behind the phaco tip as the last piece is removed can block the tip from aspirating the lax posterior capsule.

Pearls for cortical cleanup: As adherent cortex is aspirated, the usual centrifugal capsular counter-fixation afforded by stronger zonules is deficient. Lacking circumferential zonular tension, a lax posterior capsule tends to cling to epinucleus and cortex that is being aspirated, and redundant capsular folds can be easily ensnared by the aspirating instrument or snagged by a capsule polisher. While removing cortex, inadvertently aspirating the more pliant anterior capsule may cause a zonular dialysis. Effective hydrodissection is crucial because the more easily lens material separates from a floppy capsule, the less likely it is for the capsular folds to be aspirated.

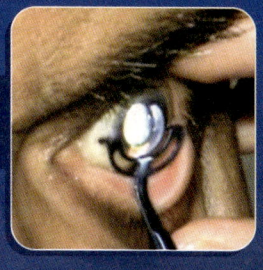

Premium IOLs (Multifocal, Toric and Multifocal Toric)

10

Pearls for Toric and Multifocal Toric IOL Implantation

Vidushi Sharma, Suresh K Pandey

INTRODUCTION

The goal in modern cataract surgery is emmetropia. Cataract surgery and refractive surgery are now seen as a surgical spectrum. With today's technology, emmetropia is easily achievable for patients with myopic or hyperopic refractive errors when the appropriate spherical lens power is chosen. Routine monofocal intraocular lens (IOLs) implantation during cataract surgery results does not overcome presbyopia and astigmatism. In addition to spherical refractive errors, astigmatism should be addressed at the time of cataract surgery so that the patient can achieve the best postoperative visual outcomes. Toric and multifocal IOLs are now available to correct astigmatism and presbyopia.

Available options for reducing astigmatism at or around the time of cataract surgery, namely performing one or more limbal relaxing incisions (LRIs), opposite clear corneal incisions, implanting an intraocular lens known as a toric IOL which corrects for astigmatism and finally postoperative PRK (Fig. 10.1). LRI technique is less precise than a toric IOL—the cornea may undergo an over-correction or under-correction. After LRI, the cornea will heal over time, altering the result. Further, the depth, length and curvature of the LRI wound will vary both within each eye and between eyes and patients, as well as surgeons.

Toric IOLs now provide a safe and predictable alternative to reduce or eliminate refractive astigmatism with a cylindrical correction, offering patients with pre-existing corneal astigmatism optimal distance visual acuity without the use of

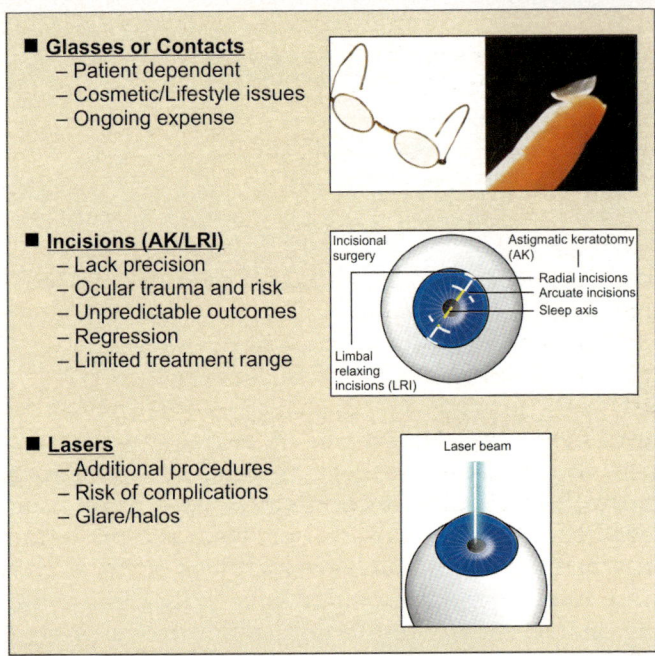

- ■ <u>**Glasses or Contacts**</u>
  - – Patient dependent
  - – Cosmetic/Lifestyle issues
  - – Ongoing expense

- ■ <u>**Incisions (AK/LRI)**</u>
  - – Lack precision
  - – Ocular trauma and risk
  - – Unpredictable outcomes
  - – Regression
  - – Limited treatment range

- ■ <u>**Lasers**</u>
  - – Additional procedures
  - – Risk of complications
  - – Glare/halos

Fig. 10.1: Treatment option for astigmatism and their limitations

spectacles or contact lenses. Approximately 22% of patients undergoing cataract surgery have substantial corneal astigmatism (i.e. more than 1.25 D) and would benefit from toric IOL implantation. This article will focus on toric IOL implantation for managing astigmatism during cataract surgery.

Currently available toric and multifocal toric IOL: At present various types of toric IOL and multifocal toric are available for management of corneal astigmatism.

STAAR surgical intraocular lens was the first FDA-approved (in 1998) toric IOL available in the United States. The STAAR toric IOL comes in a full range of distance vision powers, in two versions. One corrects up to 2.00 diopters (D) of astigmatism and the other corrects up to 3.50 D. Plate-haptic toric IOLs did not gain much preference and are challenged by poor rotational stability and a limited power range.

AcrySof IQ toric IOL (Alcon Labs, USA): The FDA also approved the AcrySof toric IOL in September 2005. Different models (T3 to T9) of AcrySof toric IOL can correct significant amount of astigmatism. This lens also is available in *aspheric* versions for crisper vision. Different models also can filter potentially damaging *UV* or *blue light*. The AcrySof toric IOL is based on the AcrySof natural single-piece platform (Alcon Laboratories, Inc.) and is a foldable lens with a fully functional, 6 mm toric optic and stableforce haptics (Alcon Laboratories, Inc.). The lens' acrylic material is highly biocompatible and has adhesive properties that, along with the haptic design, help to prevent rotation of the IOL after its implantation in the capsular bag. The posterior surface of the lens has added cylindrical power and axis markings to help the surgeon align the IOL after implanting it in the capsular bag. Online AcrySof toric IOL calculator available (www.acrysoftoriccalculator.com) to calculate the type/model of IOL (Fig. 10.3). Recently **AcrySof IQ ReSTOR toric** IOL is also available. The AcrySof® IQ ReSTOR® Multifocal toric IOL combines the technologies of Alcon's market-leading AcrySof® IQ ReSTOR® + 3 add

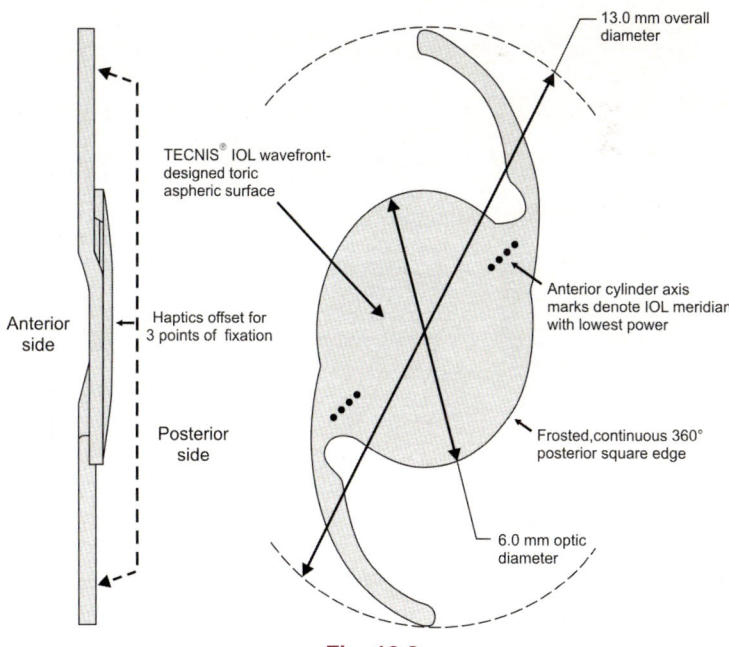

Fig. 10.2

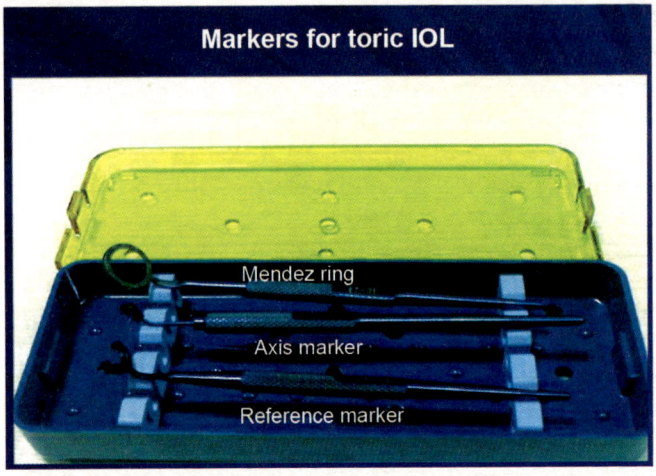

Markers for toric IOL

Mendez ring

Axis marker

Reference marker

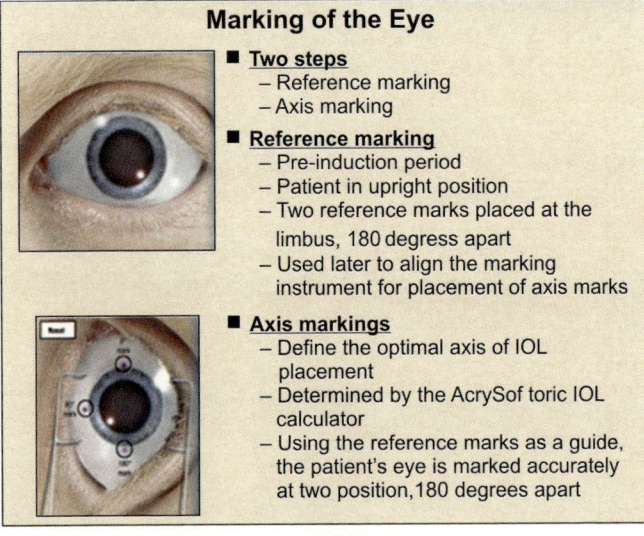

Marking of the Eye

- **Two steps**
  - Reference marking
  - Axis marking

- **Reference marking**
  - Pre-induction period
  - Patient in upright position
  - Two reference marks placed at the limbus, 180 degress apart
  - Used later to align the marking instrument for placement of axis marks

- **Axis markings**
  - Define the optimal axis of IOL placement
  - Determined by the AcrySof toric IOL calculator
  - Using the reference marks as a guide, the patient's eye is marked accurately at two position, 180 degrees apart

Fig. 10.3

multifocal IOL and the AcrySof® toric IOL. At the time of this writing, we have opportunity to implant 3 AcrySof® IQ ReSTOR® multifocal toric IOLs at our center with excellent outcome. The AcrySof® IQ ReSTOR® multifocal toric IOL have ability to deliver excellent visual outcome with independence from glasses in majority of cases.

Acri.Comfort 646TLC and Acri.LISA Toric 466TD (Carl Zeiss Meditec)

Two main models of toric IOLS: Acri.Comfort 646TLC and Acri.LISA toric 466TD marketed by **Carl Zeiss Meditec**. The Acri.Comfort 646TLC is an aspherical bitoric IOL. It was the first designed to be inserted through incisions smaller than 2 mm and so is thought to minimize the surgically induced astigmatism (SIA). Its technical features are: hydrophilic acrylic polymer containing 25% water, hydrophobic surface, plate design with square edges in haptic and optic, total diameter 11 mm, optic diameter 6.0 mm, A-constant of 118.0, spherical powers available from –10.0 to +32.0 D and a cylinder powers from +1.00 to +12 D (cylinder values outside the standard range are manufactured individually). The Acri.LISA toric 466T D is a multifocal toric IOL also designed for MICS aimed at presbyopic cataract patients with a distinct astigmatism.

Rayner T-*flex*® aspheric toric IOLs: Rayner T-*flex*® aspheric toric IOLs (573T and 623T) are a superior alternative to toric IOLs with a restricted range of torus and offer a precise, superior alternative to incisional keratotomy and limbal relaxing incisions (LRIs) for the treatment of pre-existing corneal astigmatism. With T-*flex*® aspheric toric IOLs, the torus (cylinder) is implemented on the anterior surface of the optic and the Amon-Apple enhanced square edge on the posterior surface.

T-*flex*® aspheric toric IOLs are particularly useful for those cataract patients where incisional methods would provide inadequate astigmatic correction. The choice of a T-*flex*® aspheric toric IOL leads to more precise surgical results, especially for cases of severe astigmatism: patients with a history of corneal pathology, keratoconus with penetrating keratoplasty (corneal grafts) and patients with burns and corneal scarring. Unlike plate-haptic and multipiece toric IOLs, T-*flex*® aspheric toric IOLs have inherent rotational stability. Superb visual outcomes are achieved because of the dependable absence of rotation in lenses designed with Rayner's *AVH*.

Rayner Sulcoflex toric 653T (piggyback sulcus lens): Conceived for correcting post-surgical or residual ametropia, Rayner has designed one of its Sulcoflex pseudophakic supplementary IOLs for correcting refractive cylinders using piggy-back techniques. The lens offers the following features: One piece foldable design with modified undulated chaptics; large optical zone designed to reduce the contact between lenses with round optic edge to decrease disphotopsia; customized cylinder range of +1.00 to +6.00 D in 0.5 D increments.

AMO TECNIS toric and multifocal toric IOL: The *TECNIS®* **toric** provides the stability and precision required in astigmatism correction with the proven, advanced optics, materials and design found in every *TECNIS®* IOL (Fig. 10.2).

Patient Counseling, Selection Criteria and Indications for Toric IOL

The marking procedure is done in two steps by using currently available marking kits.

First, the surgeon places reference marks at the 3 and 9 o'clock meridians at the limbus, either in the OPD room or in the OR. This step should be done with the patient sitting upright to avoid the effect of cyclorotation when the patient moves to a supine position for the cataract procedure. The surgeon then performs a standard capsulorhexis, hydro-dissection, and phacoemulsification. After cataract removal, using the reference marks, the surgeon places axis marks to delineate the steep axis of astigmatism upon which the IOL should be aligned.

Aligning the Toric and Multifocal Toric IOL with the Axis

Precisely aligning the IOL with the predetermined axis of placement involves gross alignment, viscoelastic removal, and final alignment. The first occurs after the IOL's implantation but before it has unfolded fully in the capsular bag. The IOL should be rotated to a point that is 15° to 20° counterclockwise of the final axis' location. The surgeon must ensure that the IOL does not rotate beyond the final axis during the viscoelastic's removal. It is important to remove all of the viscoelastic, including on the posterior side of the lens, because remnants could cause rotation of the IOL postoperatively.

There are various techniques and instrumentation that a surgeon may use to achieve precise on-axis alignment of the

IOL. Our preferred technique is to use an irrigation port and an IOL dialer/Sinskey hook through the sideport incision to achieve gross alignment. We then use the IOL dialer to hold the implant in place while we remove the viscoelastic with the I/A tip. Then, we use the IOL dialer or Sinskey hook once again to carefully nudge the IOL into the final alignment with the axis. Regardless of which surgical technique a surgeon chooses to employ, the precise alignment of the IOL is critical to achieving excellent outcomes with the toric IOL during postoperative period.

- The surgeon should make a small change in routine practice, by screening the patient for keratometry first and then counsel patient for cataract surgery. Patients having ≥ 1.00 D corneal cylinder are candidate for toric IOL. The counselor/ surgeon should educate patient that the technology is available for cylindrical correction. Toric IOL cases have high level of spectacle freedom for distance when implanted bilaterally (97%). The surgeon/counselor should give option to all patients having astigmatism. One should emphasize that after removal of cataract surgery their distance vision will improve (with need of using minor correction), however, they will need spectacle for near and intermediate work (reading, computer). Staff training and patient education is important.

- Proper patient selection is critical to achieve success for toric IOL implantation. Suitable candidates are cataract patients with pre-existing corneal astigmatism >1.00 D with the following characteristics: manual keratometry: steep and flat meridians ~90° apart; corneal topography: symmetrical astigmatism; during surgery: intact capsular bag compatible with continuous curvilinear capsulotomy performed with in-the-bag placement of the IOL.

- Though automatic keratometer can be helpful to take kerato-metry reading in a busy OPD, however, it is recommended to use manual keratometry and topography for magnitude, orientation, and type of pre-existing corneal astigmatism. Subjective refraction data is not advised in order to avoid the influence of any lenticular astigmatism, which will be eliminated when the cataractous lens is removed.

The surgeon should defer using toric IOL in cases of irregular corneal astigmatism caused by corneal opacity, scarring, pterigium, peripheral corneal degeneration, cases of previous ocular trauma leading to compromised capsular bag, capsular bag-zonular complex, etc.

Toric and Multifocal Toric IOL: Surgical Technique

Though several types of toric IOLs available today, we have experience of implanting AcrySof toric IOL since last 4 years. The write-up will focus on AcrySof toric IOL implantation. All cataract surgeons will quickly become comfortable with implanting the AcrySof toric IOL. Only minor modifications to a surgeon's routine cataract procedure are required for success. Areas where modifications are necessary include:

1. The IOL calculation for cylindrical power and axis of placement,
2. The marking of the eye, and
3. The on-axis placement of the IOL.

Toric and Multifocal Toric IOL: IOL Power Calculation

Selecting the appropriate lens model for a particular patient begins with determining the required spherical IOL power. Surgeons should use the method and formulae they prefer for conventional monofocal IOLs to determine each patient's spherical power requirements. The main criteria for an AcrySof toric IOL are the patient's desire for spectacle independence at distance and the presence of more than 1.00 D of corneal astigmatism by keratometry. Surgeons should begin by calculating the spherical equivalent IOL power normally with the same optimized lens constant as for the SN60AT model. The spherical equivalent powers currently available range from +6.00 to +30.00 D. After determining the desired IOL power, surgeons can use the Toric IOL calculator.

Unlike the other programs available, the AcrySof Toric IOL calculator compensates for surgically induced astigmatism. Surgeons can also customize important variables to accommodate their preferences and their patients' needs for optimized outcomes. The toric IOL calculator requires only a few easy data-input variables (Fig. 10.3). First, surgeons enter basic information such as their name, the patient's name, and the operative eye. Second, they input data from manual keratometry (the flat and steep K reading in diopters and the meridian) and biometric results (IOL spherical power as determined by the surgeons' preferred formula). Finally, surgeons enter the estimated surgically induced cylinder and the location of the cataract surgery incision.

Next, the calculator uses the input information to identify the model of toric IOL and spherical equivalent power that is best for each patient. In addition, it determines the optimal axis placement of the lens within the capsular bag. Vector analysis compensates for surgically induced astigmatism in the calculation of IOL power and optimal axis location.

A vector is any measurement that has both magnitude and direction. For example, +2.00 D of corneal astigmatism at an axis of 135° is a vector quantity. Many surgeons do not consider the potential of clear corneal cataract incisions to induce astigmatism. The vector of the corneal wound (depending on the incision's location, size, and architecture) invariably changes the vector of the preoperative corneal astigmatism.

If a surgeon selects the amount of toric IOL power and axis placement based on preoperative keratometry, the post-operative result may be an astigmatic angular error, even in the absence of IOL rotation. Ophthalmologists who have implanted first generation toric IOLs are all too familiar with the differences that can occur between the predicted and postoperative magnitude of astigmatism and its corresponding axis.

Because corneal astigmatism and astigmatism induced by corneal wounds can be considered vectors, they may be added together. Just as pilots may need to change power and direction to compensate for the wind, surgeons may also need to calculate a new toric IOL power and axis to compensate for wound-induced astigmatic changes.

For example, an eye with a low degree of astigmatism (approximately +1.25 D) can be corrected by a toric IOL with the steep axis at 135°. Making a single- or multi-planed temporal clear corneal incision at 180° induces about 0.50 D of steepening at 90°. Although this change may not appear significant, ignoring the subsequent shift in axis will produce an angular error of approximately 0.50 D at the corneal plane and 0.75 D at the plane of the capsular bag. These differences mean the toric power of the IOL will be off by 0.75 D.

Similarly, one might consider the results of making a scleral tunnel incision at 90° to correct +2.00 D of corneal astigmatism with a toric IOL and placing the steep axis at 135°. Such an incision typically induces 0.75 D of steepening at 180°. Ignoring the shift in axis induced by the incision would produce a residual angular error of approximately 0.75 D at the corneal plane and approximately 1.00 D at the plane of the capsular bag. This type of outcome may no longer be sufficiently precise to meet cataract patients' expectations.

Marking the Eye (Reference Marking and Axis Marking)

The marking procedure is done in two steps by using currently available marking kits. First, the surgeon places reference marks at the 3 and 9 o'clock meridians at the limbus, either in the OPD room or in the OR (Fig. 10.4).

Reference Marking (Slit Lamp)
Axis Marking (in Operating Room)

This step should be done with the patient sitting upright to avoid the effect of cyclorotation when the patient moves to a supine position for the cataract procedure. The surgeon then performs a standard capsulorhexis, hydrodissection, and phacoemulsification. After cataract removal, using the reference marks, the surgeon places axis marks to delineate the steep axis of astigmatism upon which the IOL should be aligned.

Aligning the Toric IOL with the Axis

Precisely aligning the IOL with the predetermined axis of placement involves gross alignment, viscoelastic removal, and final alignment. The first occurs after the IOL's implantation but before it has unfolded fully in the capsular bag. The IOL should be rotated to a point that is 15° to 20° counterclockwise of the final axis' location. The surgeon must ensure that the IOL does not rotate beyond the final axis during the viscoelastic's removal. It is important to remove all of the viscoelastic,

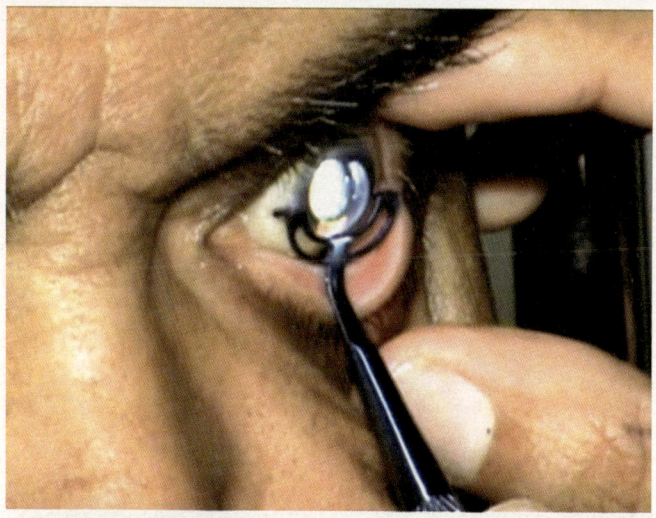

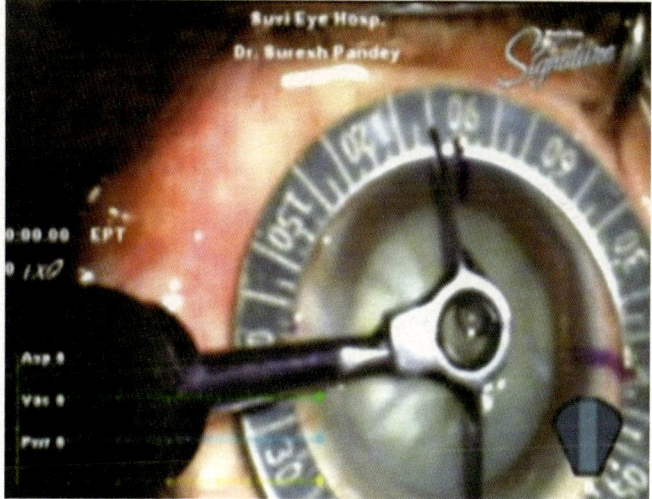

Fig. 10.4

including on the posterior side of the lens, because remnants could cause rotation of the IOL postoperatively.

There are various techniques and instrumentation that a surgeon may use to achieve precise on-axis alignment of the IOL. Our preferred technique is to use an irrigation port and an IOL dialer/Sinskey hook through the sideport incision to

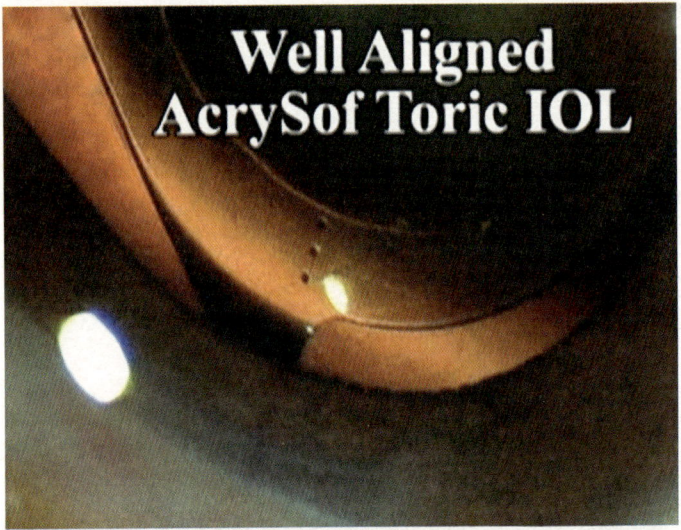

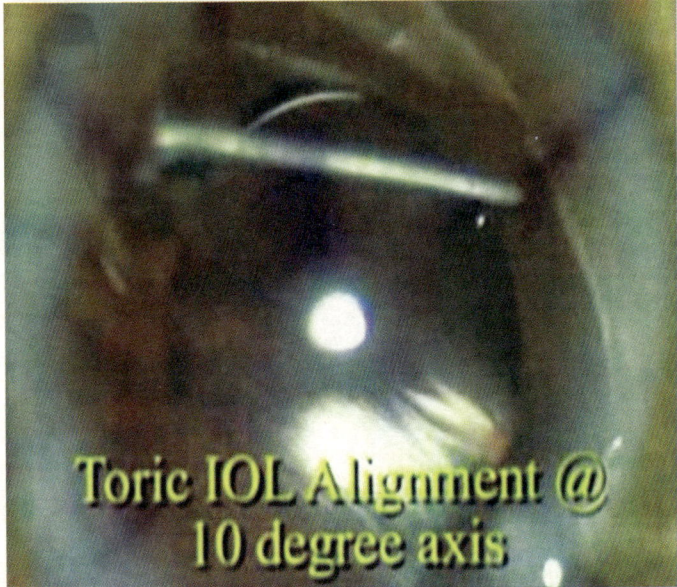

Fig. 10.5

achieve gross alignment. We then use the IOL dialer to hold the implant in place while we remove the viscoelastic with the I/A tip. Then, we use the IOL dialer or Sinskey hook once again to carefully nudge the IOL into the final alignment with the axis. Regardless of which surgical technique a surgeon chooses to employ, the precise alignment of the IOL is critical to achieving excellent outcomes with the toric IOL during postoperative period.

Surgical Outcomes and Rotational Stability

The lens must remain rotationally stable within the capsular bag to maintain its visual performance. The AcrySof toric IOL remains secure in the capsular bag as a result of the Stableforce haptic design and the adhesive nature of the acrylic material. The importance of a lens' stability and lack of rotation within the lens capsule cannot be overstated with respect to the effectiveness of a toric IOL. For every 1° of off-axis rotation, 3.3% of the lens cylinder power may be lost. At 30° of rotation, the power of the IOL cylinder is totally gone. Clearly, the axial alignment of a toric IOL determines the efficacy of astigmatic correction, and the surgical placement of the toric IOL should be as accurate as possible. During the early postoperative period, IOLs may rotate within the capsular bag until they form a bioadhesive bond with the posterior capsule. The AcrySof material allows this fixation to occur soon after the IOL's implantation.

Complications Management

An intact capsular bag compatible with continuous curvilinear capsulotomy performed with in-the-bag placement of the IOL remain extremely crucial for surgery using toric IOL. Complications with the toric IOL implantation are rare, and when they do occur, they are easily managed. One potential problem is that the implant may rotate beyond the desired axis of alignment during the removal of viscoelastic. In such cases, the surgeon can re-inflate the capsular bag with additional viscoelastic, reposition the implant to achieve gross alignment, and then proceed through the remainder of the procedure to attain final alignment. It is important to note that the lens cannot be easily rotated counterclockwise without the risk of damaging or ripping the capsular bag. Any errors in IOL power calculations or misalignment of the IOL during surgery may necessitate the IOL's repositioning or exchange.

SUMMARY

Excellent results can be achieved with the currently available toric and multifocal toric IOL with minimal modification to ophthalmologists' surgical technique. Several types of toric and multifocal toric IOLs are currently available, However, because of rotational stability and advanced IOL calculator, the TECNIS toric and AcrySof toric lens enables surgeons to correct astigmatism precisely and achieve distance-vision spectacle freedom for more patients. With availability of multifocal toric IOL, cataract patients with astigmatism can now enjoy near and distance vision with minimal dependence on spectacles. Routine cataract surgical techniques are utilized for toric IOL implantation, except accurate marking of the eye, and precise alignment of the IOL within the capsular bag.

3 Section

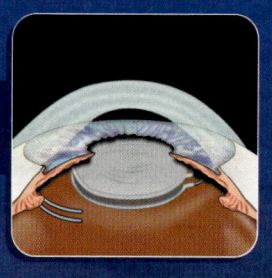

Piggyback IOL Implantation

11

Pearls for Piggyback IOL Implantation

Vidushi Sharma

Today's cataract patients expect refractive results near emmetropia and relative independence from spectacles. The surgeon therefore needs to be skilled at multiple surgical methods for correcting residual ametropia after the cataract procedure. One useful method is to implant a piggyback IOL in the ciliary sulcus over the existing lens implant. In this issue we discuss the indications, contraindications, surgical technique, and complications involved with piggyback IOL implantation procedure. Piggyback technique of IOL implantation was first described by Gayton and Sanders in 1993, this technique was initially developed to correct high hyperopic errors and as a secondary procedure to correct postoperative refractive errors. Implanting a second IOL in the posterior chamber is a relatively easy and atraumatic procedure that is not associated with the risk of potential complications seen with IOL exchange. Additionally, the accuracy of IOL power calculation is theoretically higher than in IOL exchange. Piggybacking with PMMA, silicone, or acrylic IOLs has been successful in myopic, hyperopic, and overcorrected pseudophakic patients. With the original IOL placed in the capsular bag, the piggyback IOL is traditionally placed in the sulcus in a brief procedure that takes just a few minutes. Calculating the piggyback IOL power can be done quite accurately with the Holladay vergence formula. It is also easily estimated based upon the patient's refraction. For myopic refractions, multiply the spherical equivalent by 1.2 to determine the piggyback IOL power. For hyperopic refractions, multiply the spherical equivalent by 1.5 to determine the piggyback IOL power. It is important to use an appropriate IOL for piggyback placement; these are three-piece IOLs that are made of hydrophobic acrylic, silicone or collamer material. Note that single-piece hydrophobic acrylic IOLs should not be placed into the sulcus because they may induce uveitis-glaucoma-hyphema syndrome.

Indications of Piggyback IOL Implantation

Patients with a significant postoperative refractive error have three options for its correction. The first is an IOL exchange. This procedure is best performed early in the postoperative course before the capsular bag has formed adhesions that essentially lock the IOL into place. For that reason, this option works best when the surgeon feels he or she can safely remove the existing lens implant and still preserve an intact capsular bag. Potential complications include posterior capsular rupture and zonular dialysis that can destabilize the lens implant. Another option is the implantation of a piggyback IOL, which works best in patients with a hyperopic postoperative refractive error. This form of ametropia is often less predictably corrected by an excimer laser treatment than residual myopia.

In addition to a hyperopic refractive error, the ideal patient for a piggyback IOL has a stable PCIOL that is completely

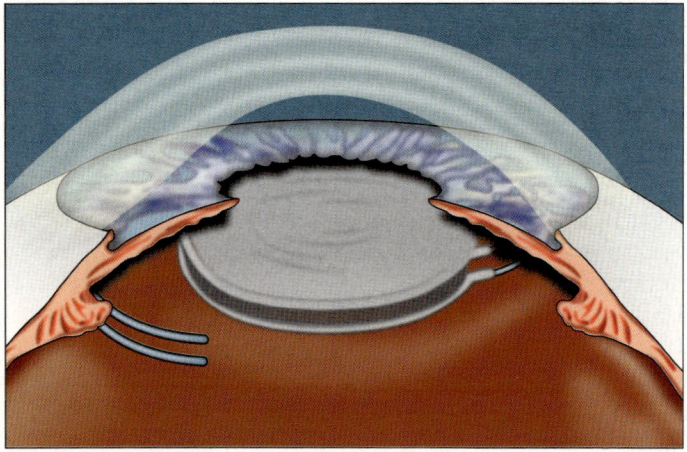

Fig. 11.1

within an intact capsular bag, a normal or deep anterior chamber, a normal corneal endothelium, and no evidence of pigment dispersion syndrome. Patients with a history of RK are also excellent candidates, because they are prone to hyperopic surprises after cataract surgery. Because corrective surgery should be postponed until refractive stability is confirmed, piggyback IOL implantation may be preferable to an IOL exchange in these patients.

Who are Less Suitable Cases for Piggyback IOLs?

Piggyback IOL implantation should be avoided in presence of pigmentary dispersion syndrome, especially in the presence of glaucoma or elevated IOP. Patients with loose zonules from trauma or pseudoexfoliation are not good candidates for piggyback IOLs. Neither are those who required a capsular tension ring for primary lens implantation. Posterior synechiae to the capsular bag are another contraindication to the placement of a piggyback lens. Patients with a significantly reduced corneal endothelial cell count are at risk for corneal endothelial cell decompensation with a piggyback IOL, but patients with mild guttata can tolerate these lenses. Piggyback lenses can correct spherical refractive errors but not astigmatism.

IOL Options for Piggyback IOLs

It is recommended that different IOL materials, in different locations, be used for the creation of a polypseudophakia lens pair. For placement in the capsular bag, an IOL with a negative shape factor such as the three-piece hydrophobic acrylic IOL is an excellent choice because at +30.00 D, all but 1/5th of the lens power is located on the posterior surface. For the ciliary sulcus lens, a large diameter, low profile, round edge, biconvex newer generation silicone IOL, such as the STAAR AQ-2010V (+5.00 D to +30.0 D) or the extended power range STAAR AQ-5010V (−4.00 D to +4.00 D) is recommended. This IOL combination lowers the likelihood of pigment dispersion, iris transillumination defects, intermittent uveitis, or secondary glaucoma, as well as the occasional "teeter tottering" of the sulcus placed IOL over a biconvex, or positive shape factor, capsular bag IOL. This also lessens the occurrence the complication of interlenticular opacifications, which has all but disappeared following the abandonment of the original bag-bag acrylic combination. Note that single-piece hydrophobic acrylic IOLs should not be placed into the sulcus because they may induce uveitis- glaucoma-hyphema syndrome.

The Sulcoflex Pseudophakic Supplementary IOL

The Sulcoflex (Rayner Intraocular Lenses Ltd., East Sussex, United Kingdom) is another suitable option for piggyback IOL. The Sulcoflex is a one-piece hydrophilic acrylic IOL with a 6.5 mm optic and 13.5 mm overall length. The optic has a round edge with a concave posterior surface and convex anterior surface. The haptics have 10° posterior angulation. These characteristics ensure separation of the IOL from the iris anteriorly, and the primary IOL posteriorly, resulting in significant reduction in the risks of ILO and iris chafing. The Sulcoflex can be used to correct pseudophakic spherical ametropia, pseudophakic astigmatic ametropia, or pseudophakic presbyopia.

Piggyback IOL: How to Calculate IOL Power?

Piggyback IOLs produce accurate refractive results. Unlike with an IOL exchange, the lens power calculations rely entirely on the patient's pseudophakic refractive error. The only data necessary for a proper IOL calculation is the A-constant of the piggyback IOL and the postoperative pseudophakic refractive spherical equivalent. For patients with postoperative hyperopic refractive errors, the spherical equivalent is multiplied by 1.5 to calculate the proper piggyback IOL power. For myopic refractive errors, the spherical equivalent is multiplied by 1.2 to calculate the necessary myopic piggyback IOL power.

Surgical Technique for Piggyback IOL Implantation

The implantation of a piggyback IOL is technically easy. The foldable IOLs can be inserted through a 2.6 mm incision. We load the piggyback IOL into the injector and fill the anterior chamber with a dispersive viscoelastic (Alcon Viscoat) to protect the corneal endothelium. Next, distend the ciliary sulcus space using a cohesive viscoelastic and then slowly inject the implant into the eye using an IOL injection system. The lead haptic can initially be placed directly into the ciliary sulcus, or the entire lens may be placed in the anterior chamber. We then insert the trailing haptic into the eye and tuck it under the iris using either a Kelman-McPherson forceps or a Sinskey hook. If the lens was initially delivered completely into the anterior chamber, we place both haptics under the iris using a hook. Ideally, there will be a slight separation between the IOL that is fixated in the bag and the piggyback IOL that is fixated in the sulcus. There should also be some space between the anterior aspect of the piggyback IOL and the undersurface of the iris. When the piggyback IOL is in a stable position, we remove all of the viscoelastic from the eye. The corneal incision can either be closed using stromal hydration or a suture. Fortunately, the surgical technique for piggyback IOL implantation is familiar to all cataract surgeons and does not require additional equipment or a learning curve.

Surgical Technique of the Sulcoflex Pseudophakic Supplementary IOL

The surgical technique is fairly straightforward but warrants a brief description for the beginning surgeon. A 2.6 mm clear corneal incision is made, followed by injection of a cohesive ophthalmic viscosurgical device (OVD) into the anterior chamber and sulcus. Folding of the Sulcoflex IOL is performed under the operating microscope to ensure correct lens positioning. The lens is injected into the sulcus with subsequent careful positioning and centration of the IOL.

In the case of the Sulcoflex multifocal IOL, aspiration of OVD (including from the interface) is followed by injection of acetylcholine chloride to constrict the pupil, allowing the surgeon to confirm that the lens is centered.

Indications for iridotomy: Iridotomy is not required in routine cases but may be considered in certain circumstances, such as in short eyes or when there are unusual features that predispose to angle closure. An iridotomy may be created preoperatively with an Nd:YAG laser or at the time of surgery.

What are Complications of Piggyback IOLs?

As with any surgical procedure, piggyback IOL implantation can cause complications. They are the same as with any intraocular procedure plus other complications unique to the piggyback IOL. The most common is interlenticular opacification (ILO), which occurs when a membrane grows between the primary lens implant and the piggyback IOL. The incidence of this complication can been significantly reduced through the use of an acrylic lens in the bag and a silicone piggyback IOL in the sulcus. Two acrylic lenses or two lens implants within the capsular bag produce a higher incidence of ILO. Another complication is postoperative pigment dispersion, which occurs when the piggyback lens rubs against the posterior surface of the iris. The use of a lens with a thin profile and a smooth, rounded edge reduces the risk of this problem. Other complications include chronic iridocyclitis, glaucoma, hyphema, and corneal decompensation. Lastly, zonular disruption and posterior capsular rupture can occur if the IOL's insertion is traumatic.

We have also performed piggyback implantation of multifocal and toric IOLs in few cases of hyperopia needing high IOL power (34 diopters) (Fig. 11.2).

Conclusions

Piggyback IOL implantation is a unique solution to the problem of to treat high hyperopia but also as a secondary technique to treat pseudophakic refractive errors to avoid the risks associated with lens exchange. With the advent of minus-power IOLs, multifocal and toric Sulcoflex IOL, the technique can benefit even myopic pseudophakes and those desires less dependence on reading glasses. Secondary piggyback implantation is helpful for patients who have had a corneal refractive procedure and are thus more likely to have postcataract surgery refractive error. Secondary piggybacks also can be used to correct the often high refractive errors of pseudophakic penetrating keratoplasty (PK) patients, for whom lens exchange presents even more risk.

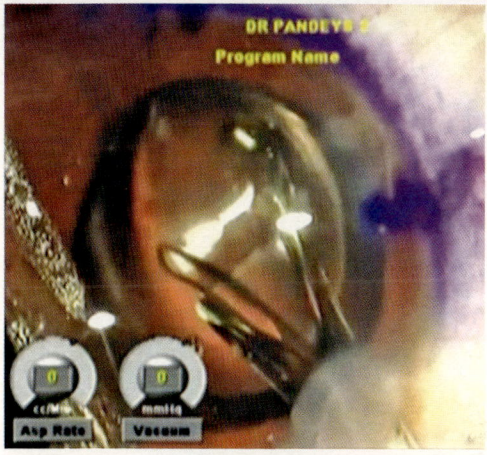

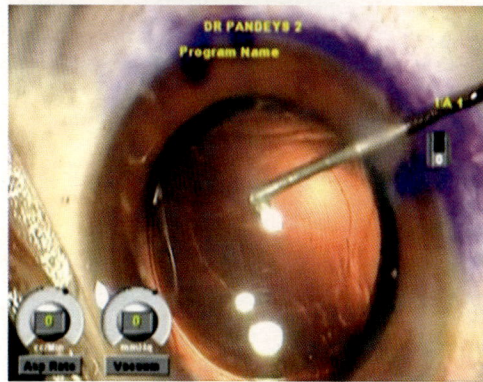

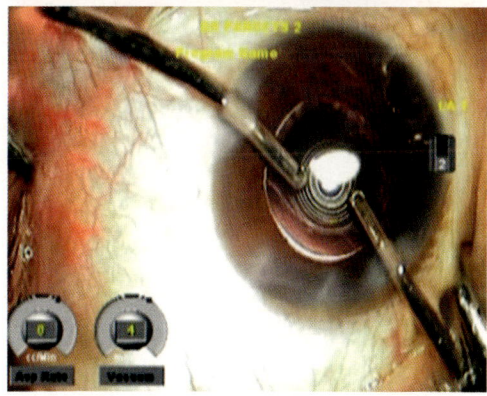

Fig. 11.2

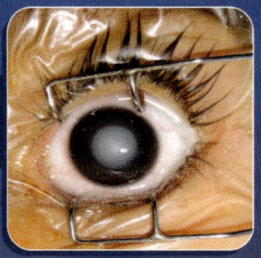

Pediatric Cataract Surgery

12

Management of Congenital/Infantile Cataract

Suresh K Pandey

Cataract surgery in children for congenital cataract remains complex and challenging and a correct management is essential to prevent permanent visual loss. Managing cataract in children need a team effort and this team consists of ophthalmologist, pediatrician, anesthetist and parents/family members. Decreased scleral rigidity and increased vitreous up-thrust make surgical manipulations within these eyes more difficult. The anterior chamber is often unstable; the capsule management requires special considerations and the propensity for postoperative inflammation is increased. Ocular growth makes selection of an intraocular lens power difficult. Normal childhood behavior can make compliance with postoperative instructions difficult, and examinations of the eye after surgery are also often challenging. The long expected life span after surgery for children also deserves consideration when surgical decisions are made. A propensity for increased postoperative inflammation and capsular opacification, a refractive state that is constantly changing due to growth of the eye, difficulty in documenting anatomic and refractive changes due to poor compliance, and a tendency to develop amblyopia are among the factors that make the cataract surgery in the child different from that in the adult (Fig. 12.1).

The aim of congenital cataract surgery is to provide and maintain a clear visual axis and a focused retinal image. The long-term visual outcome is often negatively affected by the development of amblyopia secondary to the cataract itself, or due to postoperative re-opacification of the ocular media. This write highlights surgical pearls for managing congenital cataracts and

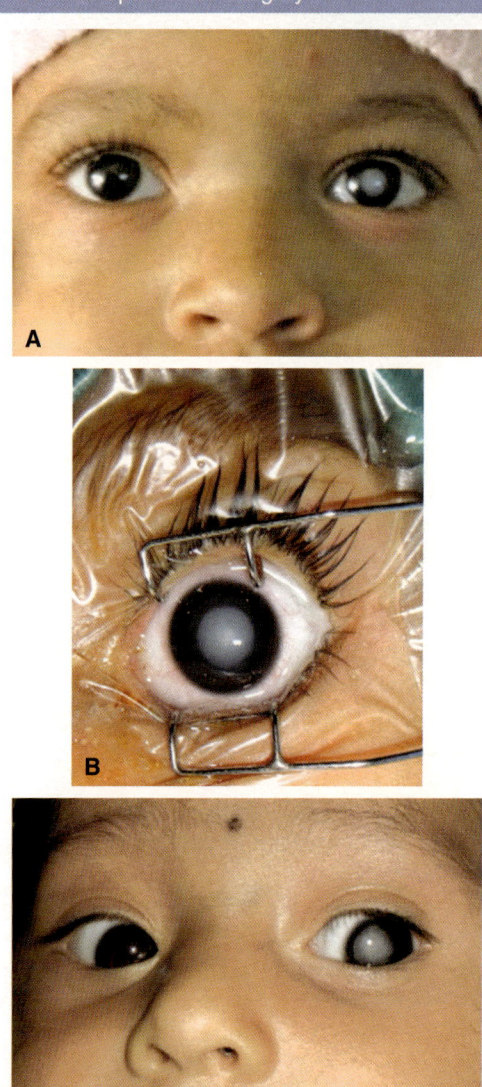

Fig. 12.1(A, B, C): *Examples of visually significant congenital cataract in infants referred to our center for management. Visually significant in children with unilateral cataract can operated as early as 4 weeks (1 month) of age. Visually significant bilateral cataract can be taken for surgery by 6 weeks of age. In bilateral cases, the surgery should be planned 1 week apart to avoid development of amblyopia*

also serves as step-by-step approach for congenital cataract surgery in general anesthesia, based on author's experience managing these cases at our facility, SuVi Eye Institute and Lasik Laser Center, Kota, Rajasthan, India (Fig. 12.2).

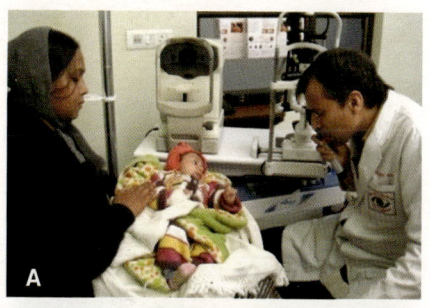

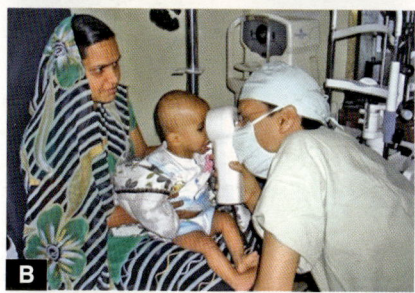

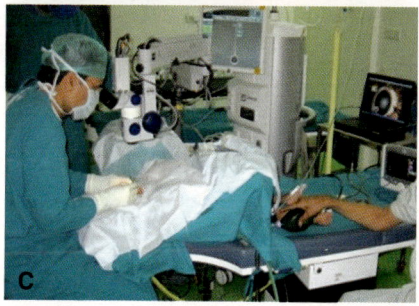

Fig. 12.2(A, B, C): *Preoperative examination (IOP, thorough anterior and posterior segment evaluation) of children with congenital cataract should be done while examination under anesthesia (EUA). However, the ophthalmologist should never miss the opportunity to examine children with congenital cataract in OPD set up when child is comfortable in mother's lap. (A) Distant direct ophthalmoscopy to assess visually significant cataract; (B) Keratometry (K reading) using hand-held keratometer; and (C) Congenital cataract surgery performed in general anesthesia*

Congenital Cataract Surgery: Counseling

As mentioned before, managing cataract in children need a team effort and this team consists of ophthalmologist, pediatrician, anesthetist, counselor and parents/family members. Before surgery, the pediatric counselor should spend time with parents/family members explaining the need for regular follow up, examination under anesthesia, need for using glasses, and compliance with amblyopia therapy. The parents should be encouraged to ask questions and clarify doubts if they have any. It may be helpful to provide parents/family members to go through patient information literature (printed in Hindi/local language) so they can understand about the disease itself and line of management.

Congenital Cataract Surgery: Indications for Surgery

The surgery is indicated for children presenting with visually significant cataract that includes: lenticular opacity in central visual axis, bigger than 3 mm; posterior cataract, opacity with no clear zones in between, when retinal details not visible with direct ophthalmoscope, nystagmus or strabismus present, or the child has poor central fixation after 8 weeks.

Congenital Cataract Surgery: Timing of Surgery

Cataract surgery and intraocular lens implantation for visually significant cataract. **Visually significant in children with unilateral cataract can operated as early as 4 weeks (1 month) of age. Visually significant bilateral cataract can be taken for surgery by 6 weeks of age.** In bilateral cases, the surgery should be planned 1 week apart to avoid development of amblyopia. Children with non-visually significant cases should be followed up regularly.

Congenital cataract surgery: Preoperative and intraoperative medications

1. *Topical antibiotic:* We prefer using the antibiotic drop (4th generation fluoroquinolone, Vigamox, Alcon Lab., USA) every 15 minutes (4 times) on the day of surgery.
2. *The dilating drops:* We prefer diluted dilator drops {5% phenylephrine, 0.5% tropicamide} in children less than 6 years are also given every 15 minutes (3 times).

3. 0.5 mL epinephrine 1:1000 solution should be added to the 500 mL bottle of irrigating solution.

Congenital cataract surgery: Pearls for incision construction: Children have thin sclera and, as mentioned above, markedly decreased scleral rigidity when compared with adults. Scleral collapse results in increased positive vitreous pressure (called "vitreous up-thrust" by some). Collapse of the anterior chamber is much more common when operating on pediatric eyes. Pediatric cataracts can be removed through a relatively small wound, as the lens has no hard nucleus. Therefore, wounds should be constructed to provide a snug fit for the instruments that pass into the anterior chamber. These incisions should not be larger than necessary for the instruments being used. For instance, a microvitreoretinal (MVR) blade can be used that creates a 20-gauge opening for a 20-gauge vitrector/aspirator to enter the anterior chamber. A 20-gauge blunt tipped irrigating cannula can also be used through a separate MVR blade stab incision. If the instrument positions need to be reversed, the snug fit is maintained. If 23 gauge or 25 gauge instruments are used, an MVR for that gauge opening can be utilized. While some surgeons prefer phaco-aspiration (aspiration utilizing a standard phacoemulsification handpiece), we prefer bimanual technique using an irrigating handpiece and a separate aspiration handpiece. Anterior chamber stability is maintained by limiting wound leak and using a high irrigation setting.

When a foldable IOL is being implanted (as in most cases today), a corneal tunnel is preferred since it leaves the conjunctiva undisturbed. The corneal tunnel should begin near the limbus for maximum healing and should be sutured with a synthetic absorbable suture. We prefer to use a marked caliper to outline the dimensions of the tunnel and utilize an angled crescent blade to make a groove and then a tunnel. The blade is turned up on its end to make the groove and then turned over to continue the tunnel.

Unlike adults, tunnel incisions do not usually self-seal in children. We attribute the poor self-sealing to low scleral rigidity resulting in fish mouthing of the wound leading to poor approximation of the internal corneal valve to the overlying stroma. The recommended closure material is a 9–0/10–0 synthetic absorbable (Vicryl) suture.

In the rare occasions when a rigid IOL is being implanted, a scleral tunnel wound is usually utilized. A half thickness scleral incision is made initially approximately 2 or 2.5 mm from the limbus and dissected into clear cornea. It is enlarged to the size necessary for IOL insertion. Closure is recommended using a 10–0 synthetic absorbable suture.

Congenital cataract surgery: Pearls for anterior capsulotomy: The anterior capsule is highly elastic in the pediatric patient and poses challenges in the creation of the capsulotomy. While a manual continuous curvilinear capsulorhexis (CCC) is ideal for adults, it is more difficult to perform in young eyes. When performing a manual CCC in a child, the following technical recommendations are offered (interested readers can view the video on following link: ttp://www.youtube.com/watch?v=jtmx5Kc-9Xg):

1. Use of an ophthalmic-viscosurgical-device (OVD) which has high viscosity (e.g. Healon5®, Abbott Medical Optics, Santa Ana, CA, USA) to fill the anterior chamber and flatten the anterior capsule. A slack anterior capsule will be easier to tear in a controlled fashion.

2. Re-grasp the capsulorhexis edge frequently and begin with a smaller capsulotomy than desired. Because of the elasticity, the opening will be larger than it appears once the forceps release the capsule flap.

3. Force when tearing must often be directed more toward the center of the pupil in order to control the turning of the CCC edge along a circular path.

4. If the capsule begins to extend peripherally, stop before the edge is out of sight under the iris. Converting to a vitrector cut capsulotomy or a radiofrequency diathermy capsulotomy is recommended when this occurs. Using a small incision capsulorhexis forceps will allow conversion to vitrector instruments when needed without leakage around the vitrector handpiece during use.

Manual CCC is most commonly used method to perform CCC in infants and children. Alternative anterior capsulotomy methods include vitrectorhexis and anterior capsulotomy using Kloti radiofrequency endodiathermy and the Fugo plasma blade.

We prefer "Ultimate soft-shell technique (USST)" for anterior capsulorhexis in pediatric white cataract (Fig. 12.3). Healon5® (Abbott Medical Optics, Inc. [AMO], Santa Ana, Calif.) and balanced salt solution are used as part of the USST to facilitate the cataract procedure and enhance its safety. After coating the corneal endothelium with dispersive viscoelastic (Alcon Viscoat), the cohesive viscoadaptive agent (Healon-5) fills the anterior chamber, thereby pressurizing the eye and protecting the corneal endothelial cells. Balanced salt solution is used below the viscoadaptive agent, away from the incision, and creates a surgical operating space with low viscosity. Anterior capsule staining is done using trypan blue by gently "painting" the anterior capsule. This, in turn, makes capsulorrhexis, hydrodissection and later, Healon5 removal, much easier.

Congenital cataract surgery: Pearls for lens substance aspiration (phacoaspiration): Pediatric cataracts are soft but they may be "gummy." Phacoemulsification is not needed and

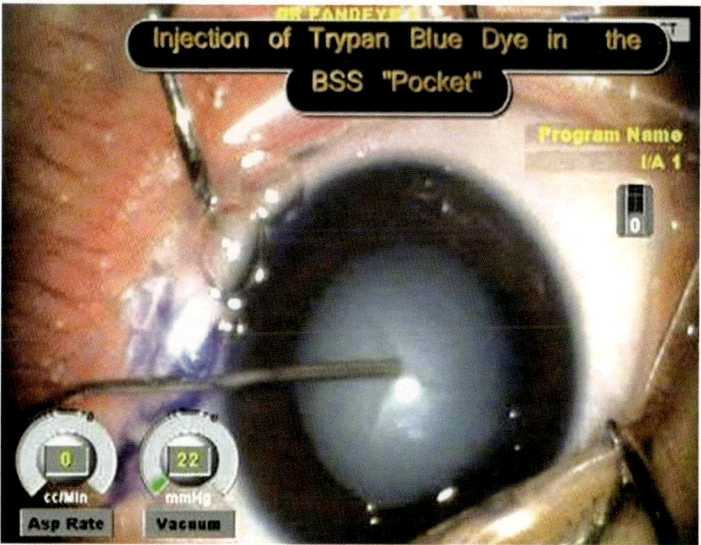

Fig. 12.3: *Congenital cataract surgery: Anterior capsule staining using "ultimate soft shell technique"*

may be harmful in the setting of chamber instability. Lens cortex and nucleus can be aspirated in every case with an irrigation/aspiration or vitrectomy handpiece (Fig. 12.4). When using the vitrector, bursts of cutting can be used intermittently to facilitate the aspiration of the more "gummy" cortex of young children. The phacoemulsification handpiece can also be used when aspirating pediatric lens material if the surgeon is more comfortable with this instrument. The benefits of hydrodissection in children are: overall reduction in the operative time, and the amount of irrigating solution used and facilitation of lens substance removal. A fluid wave can sometimes be generated in older children but not reliably in infants and toddlers. Cortical material strips easily from the pediatric capsule even in the absence of hydrodissection. Attempts at hydrodelineation should be discouraged in children since it does not aid in lens removal and may lead to capsular rupture. Posterior polar cataracts in children are contraindicated to hydrodissection because of fragility in the posterior capsule.

Congenital cataract surgery: Pearls for posterior capsule management: The advent of vitreous suction cutting devices for removing the center of the posterior capsule and a portion

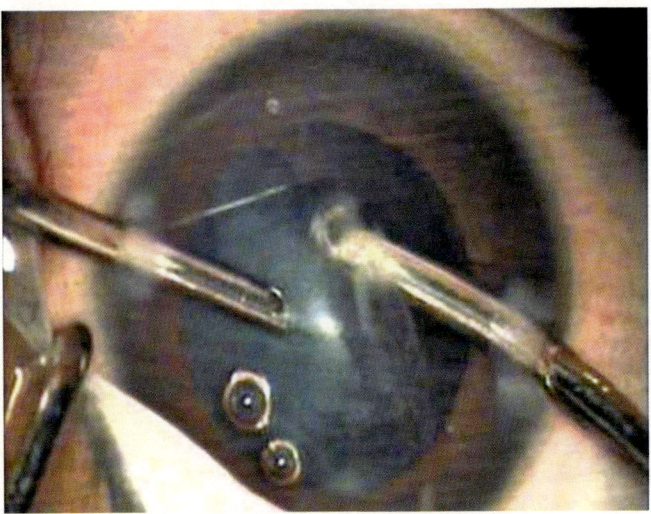

Fig. 12.4: *Bimanual irrigation and aspiration of a soft congenital cataract*

of the anterior vitreous during the initial surgery in young children undergoing cataract surgery dramatically decreased the need for secondary surgery. A primary posterior capsulotomy and anterior vitrectomy during IOL implantation in the pediatric cataract gives the best chance for maintaining a long-term clear visual axis. Neodymium:yttrium-aluminum garnet (Nd:YAG) laser posterior capsulotomies are usually necessary in children when the posterior capsule is left intact. Larger amounts of laser energy are often needed as compared to adults, and the posterior capsule opening may close, requiring repeated laser treatments or a secondary pars plana membranectomy.

Primary posterior capsulectomy and anterior vitrectomy is common practice while managing younger children with cataract. Anterior segment surgeons are often more accustomed to, and more comfortable with, a limbal (or anterior) approach. An important question that remains is, when should the posterior capsule be left intact? We answer this question looking at several factors (age, association of posterior capsule plaque or defect, availability of YAG laser, expected cooperation of child approximately 12–24 months after cataract surgery for YAG).

As a rough guideline, in children below 5 years of age, we prefer to do primary posterior capsulectomy and vitrectomy. In children, 5–8 years of age, we will do a posterior capsulectomy with or without vitrectomy, as needed. In children, above 8 years of age, we keep an intact posterior capsule more often.

Congenital cataract surgery: Primary IOL implantation: General consensus exists that IOL implantation is appropriate for most older children undergoing cataract surgery. In contrast, the advisability of IOL implantation during first year of life is still being questioned. It is well known that the majority of the eye's axial growth occurs during the first two years of life. This rapid eye growth makes selection of an IOL power for an infant difficult.

When placing an IOL in a child's eye, in-the-bag implantation is strongly recommended. Care should be taken to avoid asymmetrical fixation with one haptic in the capsular bag and the other in the ciliary sulcus. This can lead to decentration of the IOL. In contrast to adults, dialing of an IOL into the capsular bag can be difficult in children. Often the IOL will dial out of the capsular bag rather than into it. This tendency can be blunted somewhat by the use of highly viscous OVDs. Foldable hydrophobic acrylic IOLs are used increasingly in children. We prefer to implant one-piece IOL (e.g. AMO TECNIS® IOL, Alcon AcrySof® IQ IOL) that is especially suited for small soft eyes and can be inserted into the capsular bag with ease (Fig. 12.5).

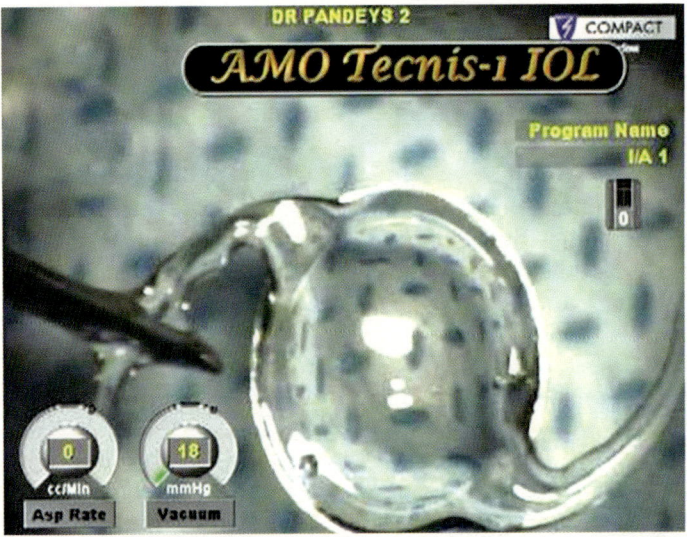

Fig. 12.5: *AMO TECNIS® one piece IOL is especially suited for small soft eyes of infants undergoing cataract surgery for congenital cataract and can be inserted into the capsular bag with ease*

When capsular fixation is not possible, sulcus placement of an IOL in a child is acceptable. To avoid decentration, when a foldable lens (such as the 3-piece AcrySof® IOL/AMO Sensar®) is used, optic capture through the anterior or combined anterior/posterior capsulorhexis should be attempted.

Toric IOL Implantation in Congenital (Pediatric) Cataract Surgery

Different models (T3 to T9) of AcrySof toric IOL can correct significant amount of astigmatism. This lens also is available in *aspheric* versions for crisper vision. Different models also can filter potentially damaging *UV* or *blue light*. The AcrySof toric IOL is based on the AcrySof natural single-piece platform (Alcon Laboratories, Inc.) and is a foldable lens with a fully functional, 6 mm toric optic and Stableforce haptics (Alcon Laboratories, Inc.). The lens' acrylic material is highly biocompatible and has adhesive properties that, along with the haptic design, help to prevent rotation of the IOL after its implantation in the capsular bag. The posterior surface of the lens has added cylindrical power and axis markings to help the surgeon align the IOL after implanting it in the capsular bag.

Recently **AcrySof IQ ReSTOR toric** IOL is also available (Fig. 12.6). The AcrySof® IQ ReSTOR® multifocal toric IOL combines the technologies of Alcon's market-leading AcrySof® IQ ReSTOR® plus 3 add multifocal IOL and the AcrySof® toric IOL. The AcrySof® IQ ReSTOR® multifocal toric IOL combines the technologies of Alcon's market-leading AcrySof® IQ ReSTOR® plus 2.5, plus 3 add multifocal IOL and the AcrySof® toric IOL. The AcrySof® IQ ReSTOR® Multifocal Toric IOL have

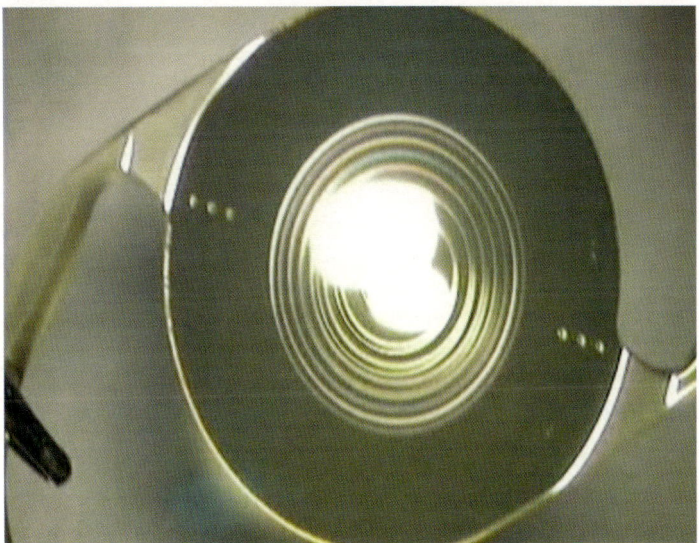

Fig. 12.6: *AcrySof® IQ ReSTOR® toric IOL has ability to deliver excellent visual outcome with independence from glasses in majority of cases. We have opportunity to implant 2 AcrySof® IQ ReSTOR® multifocal toric IOL in 8 and 10 years old children at our center with excellent outcome*

ability to deliver excellent visual outcome with independence from glasses in majority of cases. At the time of this writing, we have opportunity to implant 2 AcrySof® IQ ReSTOR® Multifocal toric IOL in 8 and 10 years old children at our center with excellent outcome (Fig. 12.7).

Congenital cataract surgery: IOL power selection: IOL power calculation in young children should be done while examination under anesthesia (Fig. 12.8). Selecting the best IOL power to implant in a growing child presents unique challenges. While Gordon and Donzis have documented the axial growth pattern of normal eyes in children, the axial growth of cataractous eyes is different. In the normal phakic child, there is little change in refraction (0.9 diopters from birth through adulthood on average) because the power of the natural lens decreases dramatically as the eye grows axially. However, an IOL placed in a child's eye cannot change in power to match the growth of the eye. An IOL chosen for emmetropia in early childhood is likely to leave the patient highly myopic in adulthood. When operating on children between the ages of 2 and 8 years, many surgeons have advised selecting an IOL power that will leave mild to moderate hyperopia, leaving less hyperopia with increasing age. Other authors have advocated aiming for emmetropia regardless of age when operating beyond age 2. This approach avoids potentially amblyogenic residual hyperopia but is likely to lead to the development of significant myopia later.

We follow the following guidelines for IOL power calculation during congenital cataract surgery: *For less than 2 years of children with congenital cataract, we prefer to use 80 percent of the total IOL power (20 percent under correction); for 2–8 years 90 percent of IOL power (10 percent under correction, after 8 years we implant IOL power providing full correction (no under correction).*

Role of preservative free triamcinolone acetonide in congenital cataract surgery: Anterior vitreous face disturbance may occur during performance of a manual posterior continuous curvilinear capsulorhexis (PCCC) in pediatric eyes during congenital cataract surgery. We prefer preservative-free triamcinolone acetonide (0.1 ml Aurocort, Aurolab, India)

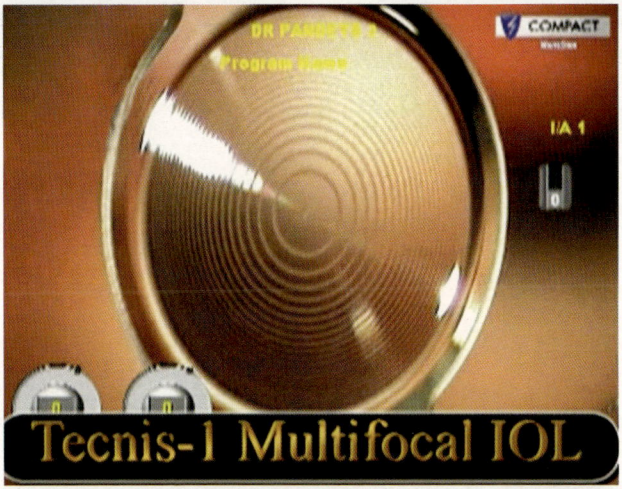

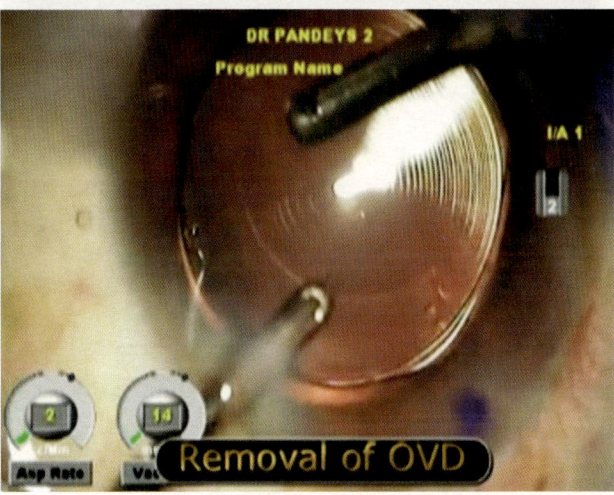

Fig. 12.7: *We have also implanted multifocal and toric multifocal IOL in pediatric cataracts more than 8 years of age and in selective cases of traumatic cataract*

suspension that appears to be effective and safe for visualizing vitreous in pediatric eyes during congenital cataract surgery, thus ensuring a thorough and complete anterior vitrectomy (Fig. 12.9). The technique renders the vitreous visible to the anterior segment surgeon and ensures a thorough and complete

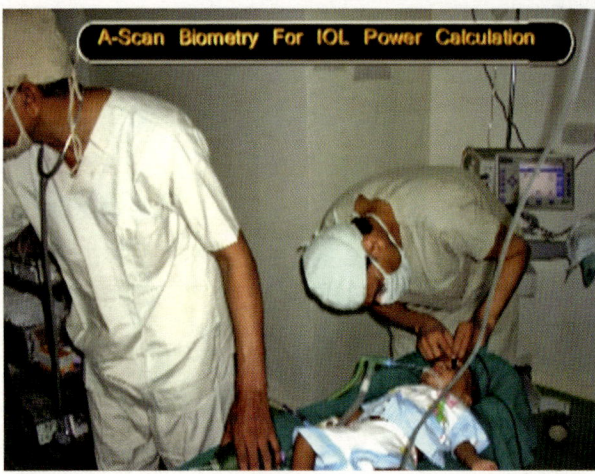

Fig. 12.8: *A scan biometry for IOL power calculation in young children during examination under anesthesia*

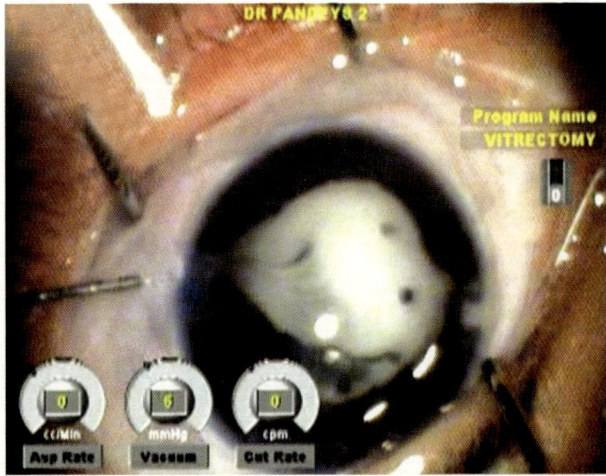

Fig. 12.9: *Preservative-free triamcinolone acetonide (0.1 ml Aurocort, Aurolab, India) suspension that appears to be effective and safe for visualizing vitreous in pediatric eyes during congenital cataract surgery*

anterior vitrectomy in congenital cataract surgery after a manual PCCC. Intracameral injection of preservative-free triamcinolone acetonide provided a safe and useful adjunct to topical steroid drops after congenital cataract surgery.

13 Phakic IOL Surgery (Implantable Collamer Lens or ICL and Implantable Phakic Contact Lens or IPCL)

Vidushi Sharma

DVD II: Phakic IOL, Lenticular and Lasik Refractive Surgery, Glaucoma, Pterigium and Oculoplastic Surgery

The latest Visian ICL model, the V4c (STAAR Surgical), with a 0.36 mm port located in the center of the optic-termed as "KS-Aquaport", which is designed to restore more natural aqueous flow and eliminate the need for an iridotomy, sets the Visian ICL V4c apart from the earlier model (Fig. 13.1), the V4b. Because we no longer have to perform an iridotomy prior to lens implantation or an iridectomy intraoperatively, the V4c is our first choice for the correction of myopia with or without astigmatism or for the correction of mixed astigmatism.

Lens Design (ICL)

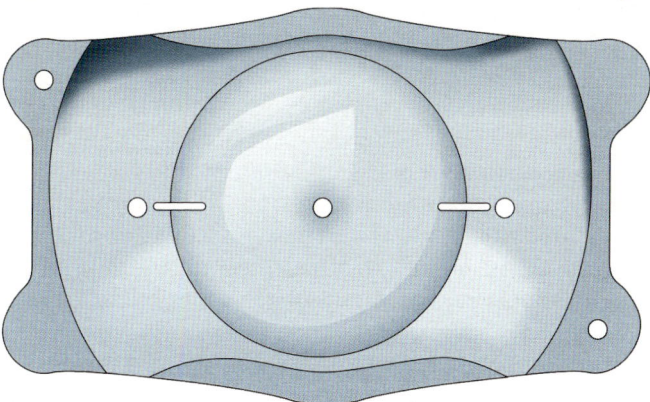

Fig. 13.1: Toric ICL: Small holes in the ICL optic eliminate the need for a peripheral iridectomy

In addition to the aquaport in the center of the ICL, the V4c also has two 0.36 mm ports located just outside the optic. Designed to simplify the removal of ophthalmic viscosurgical device (OVD) after surgery, these holes also allow aqueous to flow over a wider surface area of the crystalline lens.

Inclusion of the KS-Aquaport and the two additional ports gives the surgeon a greater safety net and patients better surgical results. Specifically, the aquaport eliminates the need to perform Nd:YAG iridotomy or peripheral iridectomy before implantation of the ICL and, therefore, eliminates the issues associated with these procedures.

Surgical Approach (Fig. 13.2)

Because the Nd:YAG iridotomy step has been eliminated with the V4c, the overall procedure is more in line with a LASIK procedure. Implantation of the V4c can be performed on the same day as the preoperative examination.

At the start of surgery, we load the V4c into an injector and fill the cartridge with an OVD. We then use forceps to pull the V4c into the tip of the cartridge until we can see all three holes. This will ensure that the lens will be delivered into the anterior chamber safely and accurately. Once the lens is in place, we irrigate the OVD from the anterior chamber, maneuvering the V4c to make space and directing the irrigation port toward the aquaport. The OVD migrates from the anterior chamber, where it can then be aspirated safely.

One day after surgery, the aquaport is still visible and can be found slightly temporal to the pupil center. Typically, the edges of the lens optic are not visible, and therefore glare is minimized. To date, there has been no induction of higher-order aberrations after V4c implantation. We have not had to change our nomogram for the lens.

In our experience, there have been no rises of intraocular pressure (IOP), no change in refractive outcome, and no patient complaints or visual symptoms after surgery (Fig. 13.3).

Conclusion

Short-term assessment of this new lens design, which incorporates a central port, showed good efficacy, predictability, and safety up to 6 months postoperative for the correction of

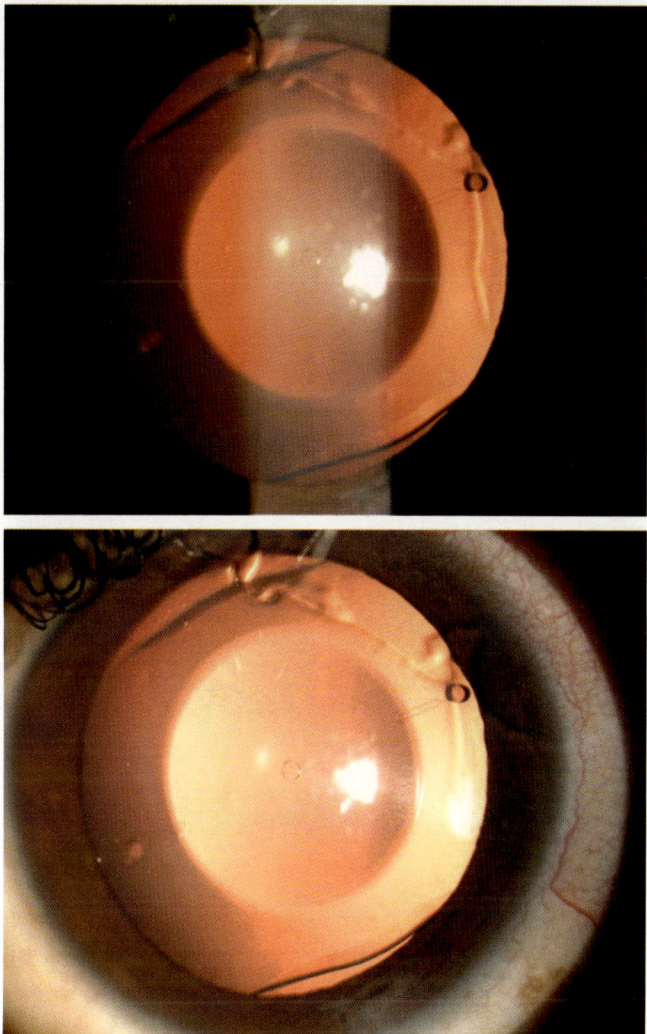

Fig. 13.2: *Surgical approach*

myopia and astigmatism. IOP was maintained and stable, demonstrating the performance of the central port.

With the Visian ICL V4c, these patients were happy with their visual outcomes, and the procedure took less time and was easier to perform than in the past. The combination of the KS-Aquaport in the center of the optic to alleviate the need for iridotomy and the additional ports outside the optic to ease removal of the OVD makes the V4c preferred choice for patients who are considering a phakic IOL.

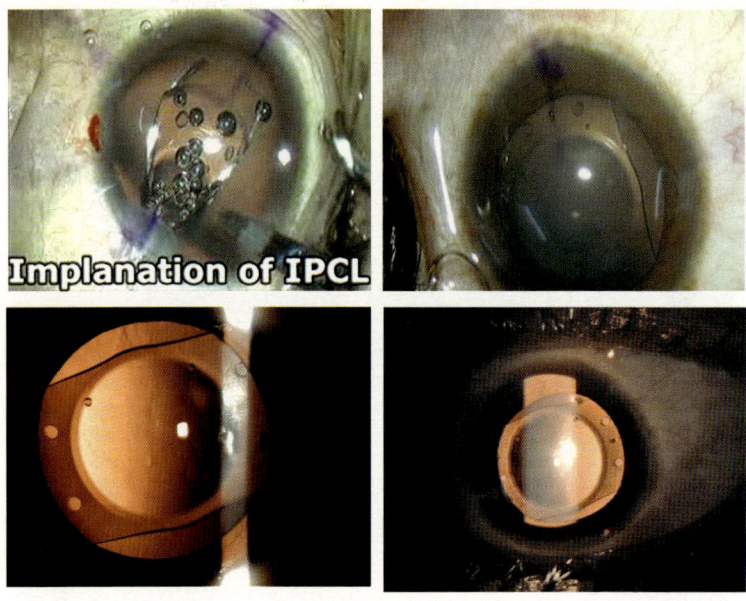

Fig. 13.3: *Implantable phakic contact lens (IPCL and toric IPCL by care group India)*

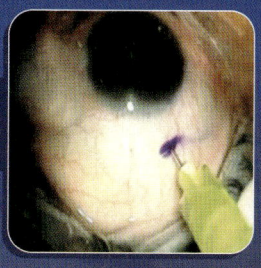

5 Section

Glaucoma Surgery

14 Trabeculectomy for Congenital Glaucoma

Pediatric glaucoma is a term that includes any form of glaucoma that presents between birth and age 18 years. Pediatric glaucoma can be either primary or secondary and the angle may be open or closed. However, there is confusing and overlapping terminology. Primary congenital and primary infantile glaucoma occur secondary to trabeculodysgenesis, a developmental angle anomaly, and can manifest any time between birth and early childhood. Pediatric developmental glaucomas are also classified by the time that they appear in a patient; primary congenital glaucoma occurring between birth and 2 months of age, primary infantile glaucoma occurring between 2 months and 2 years of age, and late onset primary infantile glaucoma (also known as juvenile glaucoma) occurring after 2 years of age. Primary infantile glaucoma overlaps with juvenile-onset open angle glaucoma (JOAG), a non-developmental glaucoma similar to primary open angle glaucoma in adults, which develops late in childhood in the absence of angle anomalies. It is most commonly accepted that the term primary congenital glaucoma refers to patients in all three age groups in the presence of developmental anterior chamber angle abnormalities.

Primary Congenital Glaucoma

- Developmental anomaly of the trabecular meshwork — trabeculodysgenesis.
- Aqueous outflow is impaired by an isolated trabeculodysgenesis.

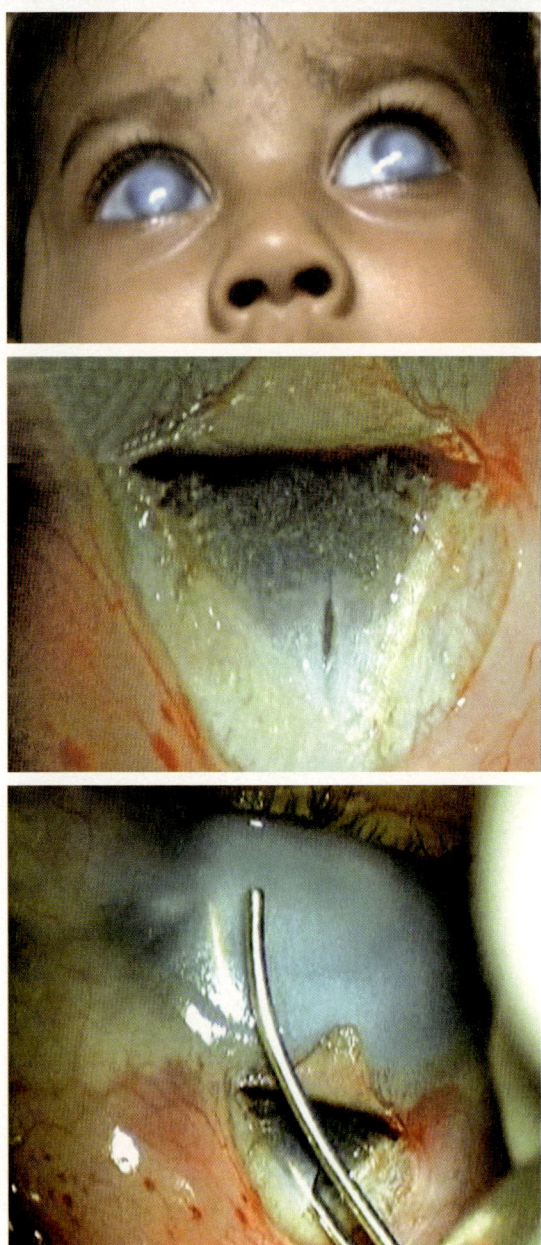

Fig. 14.1

- Maldevelopment of the trabecular meshwork, including the iridotrabecular junction, with no other major ocular abnormalities.
- Characterized by absence of the angle recess with the iris inserted directly into the trabecular meshwork. This insertion can be either flat or concave.
- Flat iris insertion manifests with the iris inserting flat and flush at or anterior to the scleral spur.
- Concave insertion is one where superficial iris tissue sweeps over the iridotrabecular junction. The scleral spur and ciliary body are obscured by the overlying iris tissue which is either sheet like or consists of a dense arborizing meshwork.
- 75% bilaterality
- Surgical
- 90% cure rate
- Known as buphthalmos
- IOP elevated during intrauterine life
- Birth through 2 mos

Primary Infantile Glaucoma

- Trabeculodysgenesis
- Manifests between 2 mos and 2 yrs
- Late-onset primary infantile – after 2 years of age
- Overlaps with juvenile open angle glaucoma (JOAG)
- Difference is trabeculodysgenesis, which is not present in JOAG
- Thus, categorizing childhood glaucomas based upon time of onset is not as exact as by mechanism of glaucoma development.

Juvenile open Angle Glaucoma

- POAG diagnosed during childhood
- Occurring between age 3 years and early adulthood
- Pressure rise occurs after 3rd birthday, but before 16th birthday
- Least common

Other Pediatric Glaucomas

- In aphakic or pseudophakic children following congenital cataract surgery.

- Mechanism in aphakic glaucoma is unclear, but gonioscopy may reveal a blockage of the trabecular meshwork secondary to an acquired repositioning of the iris against the posterior trabecular meshwork. Also, prolapsed vitreous may block meshwork.
- There is often associated abnormal pigmentation and synechiae formation within the meshwork.
- Glaucoma can occur in a pediatric patient from a number of other causes including but not limited to trauma, inflammation, episcleral venous pressure elevation as seen in Sturge-Weber syndrome, tumor, pupil block from subluxation, retinopathy of prematurity and infectious disease.

Signs and Symptoms of Primary Congenital Glaucoma

- The classic triad of congenital glaucoma is epiphora, photophobia, and blepharospasm
- Corneal clouding from edema
- Megalocornea-corneal enlargement (> 12 mm)
- Myopia
- Amblyopia
- IOP > 20 mm Hg
- Globe enlargement
- Descemet's tears-horizontal or vertical (Haab's striae)
- Scleral ring enlargement
- Rapid cupping
- Cupping reversible if caught in time

In infants, C/D ratio greater than 0.3 or asymmetrical cupping, myopic refractive error, or enlarged axial length lead to suspicion of glaucoma.

15 Intravitreal Injection of Antibiotics for Management of Endophthalmitis

Vidushi Sharma, Suresh K Pandey

DVD III: Miscellaneous—Intraocular injections, Ophthalmic Practice Management and Career Choice for Ophthalmologists

Intravitreal injection remains very important method to control endophthalmitis. We describe pearls for preparing intravitreal injection of vancomycin and ceftazidime for postoperative endophthalmitis. The commonly recommended 1 mg vancomycin dose. Use of sterile surgical gloves and sterile drappings sheets are a must. It is essential to obtain informed

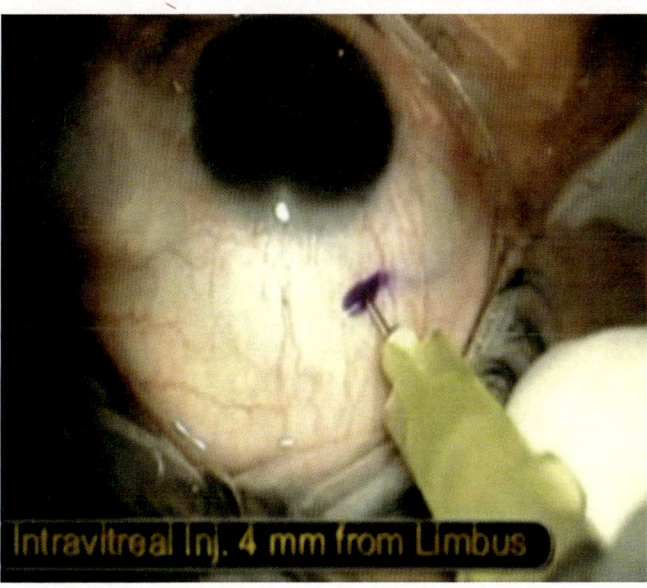

Fig. 15.1

written consent for intravitreal therapy. Scrub hands thoroughly and wear sterile surgical gloves. Prepare intravitreal injection in three tuberculin syringes based on which drugs option has chosen. The pupil should be dilated prior to intravitreal therapy.

Topical anaesthetic agents such as xylocaine or proparacaine are necessary for intravitreal therapy. However, many ophthalmologists additionally use subconjunctival anaesthetic injections at the proposed site of intravitreal injection. In endophthalmitis peribulbar anaesthetic injection is very useful, as it provides postintravitreal injection analgesia for many hours. The most critical step preoperatively, is to use 10% povidone iodine to clean the eyelids and to irrigate the ocular surface and conjunctival sac. It is necessary to use a lid speculum to ensure that the eyelashes and margins of the eyelids do not contaminate the syringe and needle during injection. Sterile gloves should be worn. Tuberculin syringes with 26 or 30 gauge needle are very useful for giving intravitreal injections. It is recommended that the conjunctiva be displaced slightly with a cotton bud prior to beginning the injection so that the conjunctival entry point is slightly separated from the scleral entry point. This allows a better wound seal postinjection.

The injection should be given 3.5 mm from the limbus in a pseudophakic eye. An attempt may be made to aspirate by gentle suction some vitreous fluid through pars plana for bacteriological analysis. Often one is likely to fail to get fluid. The needle must be withdrawn slowly letting the vitreous collagen clogging the needle to escape back without causing traction retinal tears. Take the syringe with 0.1 ml drugs. Puncture the globe at pars plana (3.5–4 mm behind the limbus). Slowly inject the content. Withdraw. Repeat the same procedure with the remaining two syringes with 0.1 ml of the solution. Please note, though it is possible to mix an antibiotic and dexamethasone, it is not advisable to mix two antibiotics in the syringe. In order that concentrated antibiotics do not settle on the Macula, one may use a pillow during the procedure and turn the head to the opposite side, immediately after the injections. After the injection the patient may maintain a face down position for 10 to 15 months for the antibiotics to move towards the anterior segment. Put a pad and bandage for at least an hour. Analgesic and a tablet of acetazolamide is optional. If improvement noted but not impressive: Repeat antibiotics and dexamethasone after 48 hours. *Definition of Improvement:* Improvement of vision, however small it may appear, reduction or disappearance of hypopyon after sitting up of 1 hour or more. Clearing of the AC, consolidation of the fibrin exudates or shrinking of the pupillary membrane, better red reflex, reduction of pain, decrease in lid edema and chemosis, if it was present, If no improvement or worsening in 48–72 hours. A repeat vitreous tap and injection of antibiotics plus a pars plana vitrectomy (if this was not originally done) should be considered. Complications of an intravitreal injection include Retinal detachment (0.0–1.0% per patient); Significant vitreous haemorrhage (0.4% per patient).

16 Intracameral Antibiotics for Endophthalmitic Prophylaxis During Cataract Surgery

Vidushi Sharma

Cataract surgery is one of the most commonly performed operations in India. Modern cataract surgery has become a safe and minimally invasive procedure that continues to produce excellent outcomes. Although the incidence of endophthalmitis is extremely low, the large volume of cataract surgeries produces approximately 4000 cases of endophthalmitis per year, with potentially devastating consequences. The basic principles of antibiotic prophylaxis are as follows:

- To deliver an active agent effective against infecting micro-organisms
- To have adequate contact time between the drug and the infecting microbe since most antibiotics require bacterial replication to completely kill of the organism
- To avoid or minimize toxicity and side effects
- To minimize the risk of developing antibiotic-resistant organisms
- To be affordable

Antibiotic prophylaxis for the prevention of endophthalmitis in cataract surgery is one of the most controversial areas in ophthalmology. This is due to the ocular morbidity of endophthalmitis coupled with the paucity of clinical studies that conclusively show an effective technique to reduce its occurrence.

Intrinsically, the concept of placing an antibiotic into the target tissue of the anterior chamber to eradicate or partially treat the potential bacterial inoculum that occurs at the time of surgery makes sense. A number of retrospective studies have suggested that intracameral antibiotics can significantly reduce the risk of ocular infection.

The ideal intracameral antibiotic would be broad spectrum, bactericidal, fast acting, nontoxic, and able to be supplemented with topical medications. Directly injecting intracameral antibiotic at the conclusion of surgery ensures that the dosage is both sufficient and nontoxic (toxicity can occur when the antibiotic is placed in the irrigating solution during a complex cataract extraction).

17

Supratarsal Injection for Recalcitrant Vernal Keratoconjunctivitis (VKC)

Vidushi Sharma, Suresh K Pandey

Supratarsal injection of steroid for resistant VKC is a new modality results in less recurrence of VKC and a dramatic and quick relief in symptoms, including itching, redness and watery discharge. Supratarsal injection of steroid is useful for relcalcitrant VKC and ocular allergy disorder and it encourages healing of shield ulcers and persistent cobblestone papillae. This relatively new modality results in less recurrence of VKC and a dramatic and quick relief in symptoms, including itching, redness and watery discharge.

Prolonged topical steroids and systemic drugs contribute to and worsen the blinding complications of VKC. Many of these patients end up in blindness from corneal ulcers, scars, glaucoma, cataract, stem cell limbal deficiencies and inadequate tear film.

Supratarsal injection of triamcinolone acetonide (Aurocart, Aurolab, India) simple and inexpensive method to treat nearly all cases of recalcitrant VKC (Fig. 17.1). The medication is easily available and the technique to administer can be quickly learned by most ophthalmologists. There is also a little risk of medication being misused because the ophthalmologist administers the medication himself.

Technique of supratarsal injection: To place medication safely in the supratarsal space, the technique has to be mastered. The conjunctival fornix and supratarsal areas are adequately anaesthetized for injection with repeated applications of local anesthetic (4% lidocaine hydrochloride instilled every minute for 4 minutes). The everted upper lid is further exposed for 1 minute with a swab stick that has been

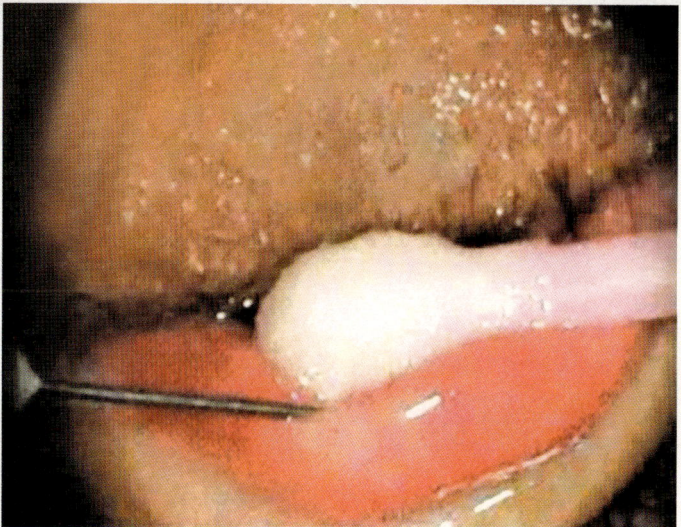

Fig. 17.1: *Supratarsal injection of triamcinolone acetonide*

soaked in 4% lidocaine. The tarsal plate is gently lifted from the globe with the swab stick and a 26-gauge needle is placed in the potential supratarsal space separating conjunctiva and Muller's muscle, approximately 1 mm above the superior border of tarsal plate.

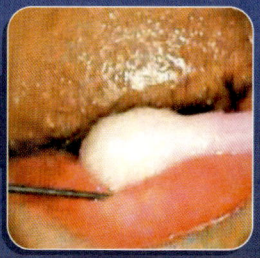

6 Section

Career Choices for Ophthalmologists Today

18

Career Choices for Younger Ophthalmologists

Vidushi Sharma, Suresh K Pandey

In the fast changing scenario of Indian ophthalmology, a variety of career choices are available (e.g. solo practice, group practice, corporate chain, academic institute in India or overseas ophthalmology) with pros and cons for each option. The ophthalmology practice patterns are changing and new forms of practice consolidations, practice merger and acquisitions, are emerging. This presentation in an attempt to bridge the gap between current ophthalmology residency and fellowship training and the requirements of starting a successful practice by choosing a suitable option.

After completion of residency and fellowship in ophthalmology, when looking for your first job, the most important thing is to be honest with yourself. What do you want? Sometimes it's hard to know. Sometimes your first job doesn't

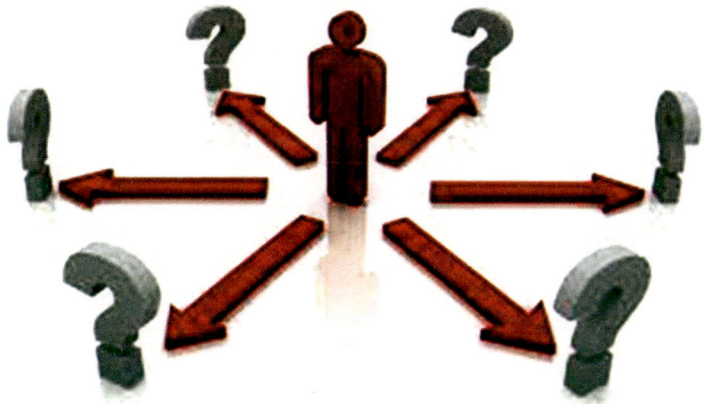

Fig. 18.1

work out because it wasn't the right fit. The more you can identify what you want to do, the sooner you can identify the right opportunity. There are a few career paths to consider:

Option 1: Private (Solo) Ophthalmic Practice: During residency, many ophthalmologists assume private practice (and eventual practice ownership) is where they're headed. Are you interested in the business side of medicine? Running a solo practice gives you freedom to run the show as you want. However, it requires lot of funds and is much more time- and energy-consuming than most of us realize.

We are running a high volume solo ophthalmic practice named SuVi Eye Institute, at Kota India and based on our experience, our advice to an ophthalmologist who decides to start a solo practice:

- *Make sure you have a way to keep surgical skills up-to-date.* In some cases, you might be better off working for a high-volume surgical practice for a while before starting your practice.
- *Be creative and flexible when buying instruments.* Sometimes new practice owners want to buy the most expensive (high end) equipment(s), but if you are starting from scratch, you will not have the patient flow to pay for this.
- *Stay in the information loop, particularly if you are a solo doctor.*
- *Be very careful with human resources issues.* It's hard to predict early on who will be an all-star and who will fizzle out. People's lives change due to divorce, health, family issues and other causes.
- *Steer away from manufacturers who try to sell you things you don't need, particularly machines that will put pressure on you financially.*

Mass communication skills and practice good interpersonal skills. You can advertise all you want, but if people do not like you and are not satisfied, they will not choose to stay with your practice. Our philosophy has always been to give great customer service and be very good medically and technically. You have to be 100 percent committed and warm and fuzzy, too. If you have all this in place, and you show up and do it to the best of your ability every day, the solo practice will definitely succeed.

Option 2: Large group practice Or corporate eye institutes: Working for a mega-practice can also insulate you from private-practice headaches. Most doctors in a really big practice just practice medicine, and do not get involved in practice management.

Option 3: Academia/research: Teaching and running clinical or laboratory research projects are intellectually rewarding and provide a setting where you can rub elbows with the best and the brightest. These jobs can lead to highly prestigious positions, and also offer the potential to help large numbers of patients by answering fundamental questions.

Option 4: Hospital positions: Staff specialists and surgeons get to practice "pure" medicine, insulated from headaches such as staff management, insurance issues, malpractice insurance, etc. When combined with teaching positions, they offer an interesting balance of professional duties.

Option 5: Pharmaceutical or medical device industry: These are corporate jobs with all the perks. A medical degree brings you in at a high level, one at which you are a critical decision-maker. You most likely would be involved with research and development of new products that have the potential to help a large number of people.

19

Greener Pastures Overseas (Career Opportunity Overseas)

Vidushi Sharma, Suresh K Pandey

Ophthalmologists who have completed fellowships abroad bring back with new ideas for improving practice and changing the way we work. Before you start looking for a fellowship, you should define your objectives and what you hope to achieve from the experience. This could be observation or improvement in a particular surgical skill, gaining teaching skills, or building international contacts. Fellowships undertaken overseas have several advantages: Experience of working in a different healthcare system with people of different cultural background can go a long way in professional and personal development and exchange of knowledge.

One can get information on fellowship opportunities from several sources, such as professional contacts and mentors; websites of specialist units and societies (such as the American Academy of Ophthalmology, International Council of Ophthalmology, etc.); advertisements on websites of specialty journals, and job advertisements in BMJ Careers. Once you have identified a potential fellowship, a serious chat with a previous (or current) fellow of the unit you intend to join is by far the best and easiest way of getting a detailed account of what the fellowship entails.

Many centers insist that fellowship candidates complete application forms to be considered for a post. However, a carefully drafted email (or letter) to the fellowship supervisor along with an updated copy of your CV is perhaps a good idea to initiate the process. Most overseas fellowships are offered only after success in a formal face to face interview, whereas

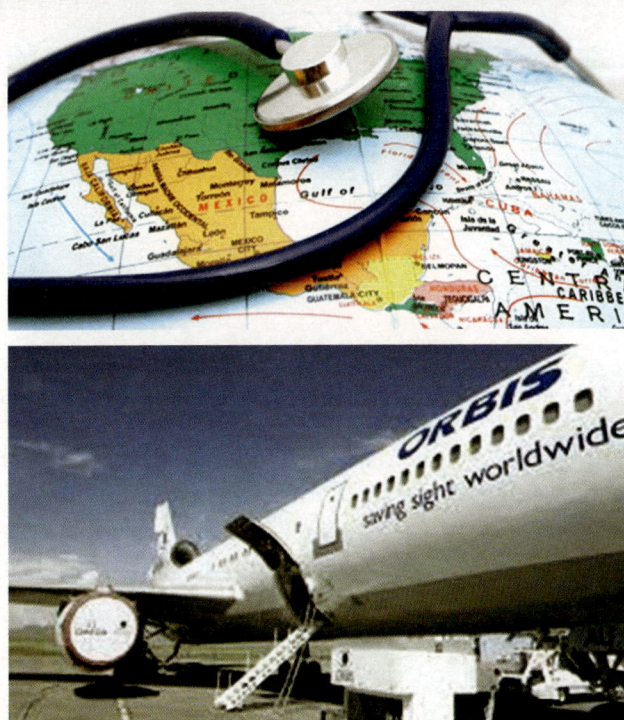

Fig. 19.1

overseas positions may entail either an informal telephone chat or nothing at all.

In preparing an application, it is important to remember that being in a training programme does not guarantee a fellowship position. The best fellowships are in high demand and attract trainees from all over the world. Although your references and contacts can help, having a robust CV in terms of publications and presentations is perhaps the most important factor that can tip the balance in your favor. Careful financial planning is essential, especially if you want to go abroad. You should have a reasonable amount of money available to cover initial and future costs.

Here is the list for pursuing a short-term or long-term training in ophthalmology:

SHORT-TERM OPPORTUNITIES (2–4 WEEKS)

University of Cape Town
Department of surgery
Division of ophthalmology
J45 Rm.69
Old Main Building
Groote Schuur Hospital
Observatory
7925
CAPE TOWN
R.S.A

The faculty of health sciences at UCT has the oldest medical school in South Africa. Its core business is research in medical and allied fields, as well as teaching undergraduate and postgraduate students over a wide range of healthcare-related disciplines. UCT offers 2–4 weeks observerships in the Division of Ophthalmology, which is under the department of surgery. Contact Professor Colin Cook, Morris Mauerberger Chair of Ophthalmology, at *myrna.colin@gmail.com* for more details.

The Fred Hollows Foundation
www.hollows.com.au (Main offices are in Australia, New Zealand and the United Kingdom)

The Fred Hollow Foundation
Level 3, 414 Gardeners Road
Rosebery, NSW 2018
Australia
Tel: 61-2-8338 2111
Fax: 61-2-8338 2100

The Fred Hollows Foundation is inspired by work of the late Professor Fred Hollows, whose vision was for a world where no one is needlessly blind. The individual offices in Australia, New Zealand and the United Kingdom formed a global network to increase their collective impact in eradicating avoidable blindness around the world. Their hope is to restore sight to over one million people. The Foundation does not generally place volunteers in their international programs because their aim is to develop the skills and capacity of local workers in the disadvantaged communities in which they serve. However, there is one particular opportunity in Kathmandu, Nepal, where eye specialists for the time being may volunteer.

Tilganga Institute of Ophthalmology
(incorporating **The Fred Hollows IOL Laboratory)**
Address: Bagmati Pul, Gaushala, Kathmandu, Nepal
Postal address: PO Box 561, Kathmandu, Nepal
Phone: + 977 1447 4685 or + 977 1449 3775
Fax: + 977 1447 4685
Email: *fhf@hollows.org* or *geoffrey.tabin@hsc.utah.edu*
Website: *www.tilganga.org*

The Fred Hollows Foundations works with the Tilganga Institute of Ophthalmology, which is an independent entity from The Foundation and has partnerships with several non-government organizations. The Fred Hollows Foundation mainly provides funding for the Institute's activities.

Led by Medical Director, **Dr Sanduk Ruit**, the Tilganga Institute of Ophthalmology is composed of the Surgicentre, the Fred Hollows Intraocular Lens Laboratory and an Eye Bank for the storage of donated corneas. Tilganga has screened nearly 1.5 million people and performed more than 74,000 operations in the Himalaya region since 1994. They have a strong infrastructure including outreach and community eye clinics, which help the Institute to achieve its vision of providing eye care services to the poorest of the poor, no matter where they live. The Tilganga Institute of Ophthalmology also provides outreach services and training for surgical teams from Bangladesh, Bhutan, Cambodia, Pakistan, Sikkim, Tibet, Myanmar, northern India, North Korea and for other country programs coordinated by The Fred Hollows Foundation.

Senior residents, surgeons and ophthalmology professors from the United States and Tilganga Eye Centre teach sections of the academic material and provide extraordinary surgery mentoring opportunities. More information can be found under the Himalayan Cataract Project at *http://www.cureblindness.org/*. The program is co-directed by Dr. Sanduk Ruit and Dr. Geoffrey Tabin (from the University of Utah). Write to *info@cureblindness.org*.

Hospital Italiano
Dr. Eduardo Mayorga
Head of the Eye Department
Hospital Italiano de Buenos Aires
www.hospitalitaliano.org.ar
http://www2.hospitalitaliano.org.ar/oftalmo/
mayorgaedu@gmail.com

El Hospital Italiano in Buenos Aires, Argentina, is a state of the art, private hospital in the capital of Argentina. The ophthalmology department receives complex referrals from all over the country and continent. They have specialists in refractive surgery, cataracts, cornea transplantation, strabismus, ocular oncology, retina, oculo-plastics, neuro-ophthalmology and glaucoma. Their residency program accepts 3 residents a year and welcome clinical observerships. Dr. Mayorga is considered one of the best in ophthalmologic education by his peers and would be willing to talk with any interested resident in creating a customized elective experience. A working knowledge of the Spanish language is highly recommended.

International Federation of Ophthalmological Societies (IFOS)
International Council of Ophthalmology (ICO)
Bruce E. Spivey, MD
President
945 Green Street
San Francisco, CA 94133
United States of America
Fax: +1 (415) 409-8403
E-mail: *info@icoph.org,*
bruce@spivey.org

Dr. Spivey is an alumnus of the university of Iowa and has graciously agreed to help residents from our program to find an international ophthalmology experience suitable to each one's objectives and goals. As President of the ICO, he has vast connections with educators from all over the world and is an invaluable resource for our community.

There are also opportunities to work directly with the ICO at the administrative level. Below is a description of the organization's history and mission.

The International Council of Ophthalmology (ICO) represents and serves professional ophthalmologic associations around the world. The formation of an international council began at the first World Ophthalmology Congress in 1857. In 1927, participants in the Congress formally founded the ICO in Holland.

The ICO's mission is to work with ophthalmologic societies, ophthalmologists and others to enhance ophthalmic education and the provision of eye care in order to preserve and protect vision for all people worldwide. Its goals are to:

- Enhance ophthalmic education, particularly training of ophthalmologists and other eye care personnel to meet public needs in developing countries
- Stimulate and support communication and collaboration among ophthalmologic societies and ophthalmologists globally and their involvement in initiatives to preserve vision
- Define and disseminate proposed standards and guidelines in order to enhance eye care
- Stimulate research to eradicate preventable blindness
- Raise awareness worldwide of the economic, social and personal impact of vision loss and advocate for increased funding and other support for preservation and restoration of vision.

The ICO produces and supports several programs including the World Ophthalmology Congress, the Basic Science Assessment and Clinical Sciences Assessment for Ophthalmologists, the ICO International Fellowship, ICO International Clinical Guidelines, advocacy for the preservation of vision, vision for the future, the international ophthalmology strategic plan to preserve and restore vision, and the research agenda for global blindness prevention. Contact Dr. Spivey if you are interested in volunteering with the ICO.

Medical Ministry International, USA
PO Box 1339
Allen, TX 75013
Telephone: (972) 727-5864
Fax: (972) 727-7810
Email: *mmitx@mmint.org*

MMI is a Christian medical mission organization whose aim is to serve God by providing spiritual and physical health care in a world of need. Their vision is to care annually for 100 million of the world's needy by the year 2050. They are committed to meeting the need for medical care among the world's poor with lasting solutions through excellence in medicine, patient care, and health education. Their strategy is to mobilize volunteers on one and two-week medical projects led by physicians with long-term relationships to the areas they serve and to establish and equip permanent medical centers.

Volunteers participating on short-term medical mission trips form the foundation of the ministry. As volunteers work hard to provide care and change lives, they, in turn, find that their lives are changed. Participants take one or two weeks of vacation time to go and minister to multitudes of people in developing countries in Africa, Asia and the Americas. Most projects are general medicine, surgery and dentistry. Eye projects may be surgical only or involve a full team of eighty including ophthalmologists, optometrists, opticians, nurses, techs, anesthesiologists, and general helpers. On their website, you can find a year-long calendar of projects.

Mettapracharak (Wat Rai Khing) Hospital

Puwat Charukamnoetkanok, M.D.
Director of International Affairs
Adjunct Assistant Professor of Ophthalmology
University of Pittsburgh
University of Illinois at Chicago
52 Moo 2
Raikhing District, Sampran
Nakornpathom 73210
Thailand
Phone: +66 34-225818
Fax: +66 34-321243
http://www.metta.go.th/ (website is not yet available in English)

Dr. Puwat Charukamnoetkanok (better known here as Dr. Puwat) is also an alumnus of the University of Iowa and is interested in hosting visiting residents and creating and resident exchange program. Anyone interested in this experience should contact him at *drpuwat@yahoo.com*.

Moorfields Eye Hospital NHS Foundation Trust
Mr. Paul Sullivan
Director of Education
Care of: Miss Jennifer Irish
PGME & Observers Administrator
Postgraduate Medical Education Centre
162 City Road
London, UK
EC1V 2PD
Phone: +44 (0)20 7566 2428
Email: *Jennifer.irish@moorfields.nhs.uk*
http://www.moorfields.nhs.uk

Moorfields eye hospital is the oldest and one of the largest centers for ophthalmic treatment, teaching, and research in the world. The hospital accepts 1–2 observers on any one sub-specialty service at one time. The following services are represented at Moorfields: the adnexal service, cataract service, corneal 7 external diseases service, glaucoma service, medical retina service, neuro-ophthalmology service, strabismus and paediatrics service and the vitreoretinal service. The minimum length of stay is 1 week and may extend up to 2 months (except for the Glaucoma service, which has a 2-week maximum). A written application and a current copy of your CV are required. The cost is 150 per week, which is due up front and is non-refundable.

ORBIS International (Headquarters)
520 Eighth Ave., 11th floor
New York, NY 10018
Tel: (800) ORBIS-US, (646) 674-5500
Fax: (646) 674-5599
Email: *info@orbis.org*
www.orbis.org

ORBIS is a non-profit organization whose mission is to preserve and restore sight by strengthening the capacity of local partners in their efforts to prevent and treat blindness. ORBIS operates the world's only flying eye hospital delivering sight restoration, education and training to local ophthalmic communities throughout the developing world. Its training program emphasizes a multi-disciplinary and multi-national approach to medicine, nursing, anesthesia, and biomedical engineering practices for quality patient care.

As part of ORBIS commitment to cultivate the next generation of ophthalmologists committed to global blindness prevention and sight restoration efforts, they have created the role of the associate ophthalmologist. This program offers a structured environment for motivated young ophthalmologists-in-training interested in international ophthalmology and/or public health.

The associate ophthalmologist serves as a volunteer member of the medical team and has the unique opportunity to network with the programs participating volunteer faculty, screen and care for patients pre- and post-operatively as well as facilitate hands-on, didactic and wet lab training sessions.

The flying eye hospital typically conducts six to eight (two-week duration) programs in any calendar year, and can accommodate two associate ophthalmologists per program week. Acceptance is competitive and awarded based on availability.

To apply for consideration and selection, each associate ophthalmologist candidate must have a degree from an accredited medical school; maintain current medical registration/licensure; be at least a second year resident, and hold a valid passport. Associate ophthalmologists will be expected to be culturally sensitive and respectful of local tradition and law.

The role of associate ophthalmologist is a self-funded position. Each candidate will be expected to fund his/her own airfare, visa, meals, and other incidental expenses. ORBIS does provide on site accommodation at the same hotel where the ORBIS team stays. ORBIS travel department is pleased to assist each associate ophthalmologist in organizing their respective travel itineraries and visa.

After residency, one can apply to be a volunteer faculty member. ORBIS requires applicants to be board certified and have a minimum of four years experience post-completion of academic training. References from two current ORBIS medical volunteers are required.

LONG-TERM OPPORTUNITIES (MORE THAN 2-4 WEEKS)

The Carter Center

Office of Public Information

453 Freedom Parkway

Atlanta, GA 30307

Tel: (404) 331-3900 Fax: (404) 331-3900

Email: *carterweb@emory.edu*

www.cartercenter.org

The Carter center's mission is to advance human rights and alleviate unnecessary human suffering. Its vision is to create a world in which every man, female, and child has the opportunity to enjoy good health and live in peace. The Carter center, in partnership with Emory University, seeks to prevent and resolve conflicts, enhance freedom and democracy, and improve health. While the program agenda may change, The Carter center is guided by five principles:

- The center emphasizes action and results. Based on careful research and analysis, it is prepared to take timely action on important and pressing issues.
- The center does not duplicate the effective efforts of others.
- The center addresses difficult problems and recognizes the possibility of failure as an acceptable risk.
- The center is nonpartisan and acts as a neutral in dispute resolution activities.
- The center believes that people can improve their lives when provided with the necessary skills, knowledge, and access to resources.

The carter center collaborates with other organizations, public or private, in carrying out its mission. In particular, The Carter center supports the River Blindness program and the Trachoma control program. Since 1996, The Carter center has been a leader in the fight against river blindness in Africa and the Americas by working in thousands of communities in 11 countries. The Carter center's River blindness program assists ministries of health to eliminate river blindness mainly through the distribution of ivermectin in the six countries in the America: Brazil, Colombia, Ecuador, Guatemala, Mexico, and Venezuela through the special *Onchocerciasis Elimination Program of the Americas* and to control river blindness in five African countries: Cameroon, Ethiopia, Nigeria, Sudan, and Uganda.

Regarding the control of trachoma, the Carter center works with its partners to implement the World Health Organization-endorsed SAFE Strategy: **S**urgery, **A**ntibiotics, **F**acial cleanliness, and **E**nvironmental improvement. The Carter center and its partners, the ministries of health in Ethiopia, Ghana, Mali, Niger, Nigeria, and Sudan, with the generous support of the Conrad N. Hilton Foundation and the Lions Clubs International Foundation, are working together to implement the SAFE strategy in order to eliminate trachoma from at-risk communities.

The Carter center offers competitive 15 weeks minimum (10 weeks in the summer) internships to undergraduate, graduate and recent students in multiple disciplines. Interested individuals may apply on their website.

Christoffel-Blindenmission (Christian Blind Mission International)
CBM/HQ
Nibelungenstrasse 124
D-64625 Bensheim
Germany
Tel: + 49 6251 131 0
Fax: + 49 6251 131 249
Telex: 468334 CBMB D
Email: *overseas@cbm-i.org*
http://www.cbmus.org

CBM (Christian Blind Mission) is the oldest and largest ministry with the primary purpose of improving the quality of life for the blind and disabled living in the world's most disadvantaged societies. They provide preventative, medical, rehabilitative and educational services to millions of people each year. CBM supports more than 1,000 projects in 113 countries, and their aid is available to all people regardless of religion, nationality, race, or gender.

CBM's goal is to find, rescue, and rehabilitate these forgotten people giving children, hope, taking whole families and communities out of grinding poverty, and building bridges between them and their communities.

The International Centre for Eye Health

Miss Marcia Zondervan
VISION 2020 Links Programme Manager
Lecturer/DCEH Course Organiser
International Centre for Eye Health,
London School of Hygiene and Tropical Medicine
Keppel Street, London, WC1E 7HT
Office telephone - 44 (0) 2079588335
www.iceh.org.uk
https://www.iceh.org.uk/display/WEB/Education

The International Centre for Eye Health (ICEH) carries out research and education to improve eye health and eliminate avoidable blindness, with a focus on low income populations. ICEH is a World Health Organization collaborating centre for the prevention of blindness and is based at the London School of Hygiene and Tropical Medicine. Courses include a 2-year masters program and diploma in community eye health and a few short courses (1–4 months). Some modules of the masters course can also be taken individually.

Kilamanjaro Center for Community Ophthalmology

Tumaini University
PO Box 2254
Moshi, Tanzania
Tel: 255 27 2753547
Fax: 255 27 2753598 I
Email: *kcco@kcco.net*
Web: *http://www.kcco.net*

The Kilimanjaro Centre for Community Ophthalmology (KCCO) was established in Moshi, Tanzania in late 2001 as part of collaboration between the Executive Director of the Good Samaritan Foundation and Vice Chancellor of Tumaini University and Drs. Paul Courtright and Susan Lewallen of the KCCO. The KCCO exists as a centre within Tumaini University's Kilimanjaro Christian medical college and is committed to

- Elimination of avoidable blindness through the integration of programs, training, and research focusing on the delivery of sustainable and replicable community and ophthalmology service.

- Building the capacity of eastern Africans to provide high quality eye services to meet the needs of their population.
- Developing internationally recognized educational programs.
- Developing a teaching and research environment that promotes health care measures beneficial to Tanzania and surrounding countries.

Every year, KCCO takes 3–4 residents, MPH students or PhD candidates. Their program is most notable for their extensive training in community ophthalmology. As such, clinical, research, and community health-related activities are readily available, however, surgical experiences are not.

Dr Paul Courtright in the co-director of the KCCO and can be reached at *pcourtright@kcco.net* if you would like to learn more about working with the program.

Operation Eyesight Universal
National Office
4 Parkdale Crescent NW
Calgary, Alberta T2N 3T8
Canada
Toll-free tel: (800) 585–8265
Fax: (403) 270–1899
Email: *info@operationeyesight.ca*
Web: *https://www.operationeyesight.ca*
This organization has some opportunities in Ghana, but they are undergoing some organizational changes and will have a more clear policy on accepting residents in 2010.

7 Section

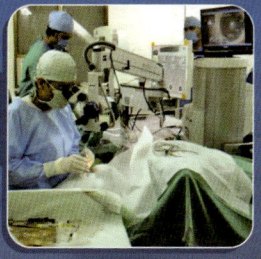

Social Media and Medical Professionalism in the Changing World

20

Social Media and Ophthalmology: Building Bridges Across the Borders

Vidushi Sharma, Suresh K Pandey

The use of social media as a special tool for medical tourism by ophthalmologists to reach out more widely and build new relationships and professional associations. These interactions can sometimes reach internationally and help in building bridges across borders in what is increasingly becoming a global village. We all know that technology has undergone a huge revolution in recent times and has also impacted the field of medical education and treatment. The place of big, unwieldy books has been taken over in many instances by slim computers and sleek smartphones. With communication becoming so fast, social media has caught on and has attracted hoards of users all over the world. These sites as well as others help us remain in touch with professional colleagues and stay abreast of the latest developments. With the availability of sophisticated and inexpensive recording and editing devices and software, surgical videos can now be easily made and shared with colleagues through various websites and social media.

REACHING GLOBALLY-CONNECTING THROUGH YOUTUBE

Our interest in documentation and sharing eye surgery prompted us to make a YouTube channel dedicated to ophthalmic surgical videos (http://www.youtube.com/user/Drsureshkpandey) which attracted many views (304, 882) and subscribers (328). This helped us to make new connections with ophthalmic colleagues, and it was our privilege to have ophthalmologists come over to SuVi Eye Institute and Lasik Laser Center, Kota, India for surgical training from as far away as Azerbaijan, Saudi Arabia, Switzerland, USA and Ireland. Their journey from a distant country to a small Indian city (Kota, Rajasthan) is a testament to the rising influence of social media interactions (Fig. 20.1).

Transcending borders: While connecting with doctors (eye surgeons) from far away is a great experience, the real adventure of social media is in being able to connect with patients and the general public. The medical profession has always moved beyond borders, an example being Doctors Sans Borders and ORBIS aircraft being another glorious example of teaching and medical services beyond borders.

Ophthalmology beyond borders: A journey from karachi to kota: India and Pakistan share a troubled border, despite many efforts for peace. Many patients, especially children, have come over to India from Pakistan to receive medical treatment as well as surgical procedures at some big institutions. However, ours is a story of a Mr Fahim Uddin, a software engineer (working at Orthopedic and Medical Institute) from Karachi,

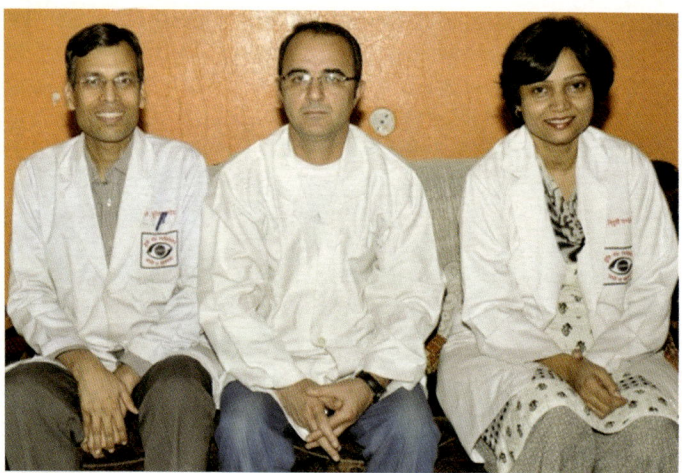

Fig. 20.1: *Social Media and Ophthalmic Training—Dr Mubariz Qahramanov, an eye surgeon from Azerbaijan visited Kota, India for a few weeks to learn and fine-tune his surgical skills in anterior segment and oculoplastic surgery. This is a testament to the rising influence of Internet, that the journey from Azarbaijan to Kota is possible despite the fact that there is no functioning airport in Kota. He watched our surgical videos on the net (YouTube) and visited SuVi Eye Institute, Kota, India*

Pakistan, who was a myope and developed cataracts at about 40 years of age. His own Internet search led him through IOL websites, and he decided he wanted a particular multifocal IOL (Tecnis Multifocal IOL, Abbott Medical Optics, USA) that was not available in Pakistan. He then searched for the IOL in India and found many videos we had posted on the implantation of this IOL. He communicated with us through social media, and, after a few interactions, developed so much trust that he decided to come to India for the surgery (Fig. 20.2).

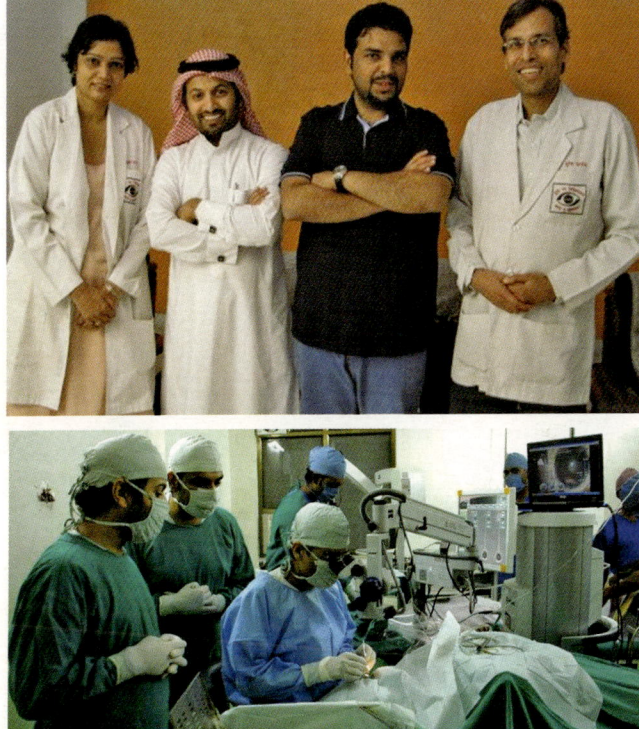

Fig. 20.2: *Social Media and Ophthalmic Training — Visiting ophthalmologists from Saudi Arabia, Dr. Hasan Al Taweel and Dr Fahad Alwadni visited SuVi Eye Institute, Kota for 3 weeks. One of the reasons they came was to observe "a small city, small set-up, without frills where you could still deliver good services in the private practice set-up"*

He came over on a medical VISA that was issued by Indian embassy in Karachi, Pakistan after thorough scrutiny. He underwent cataract surgery on both eyes with the multifocal IOL of his choice at SuVi Eye Institute, Kota and was extremely happy with the results. He even saw a Bollywood movie (*Bol Bachchan*) in the theater immediately after surgery and toured the city and was thrilled with the excellent vision he had at both distance and near without glasses, with no significant night vision problems either. The fact that he had come over from Karachi, Pakistan for his eye surgery made him somewhat of a mini celebrity, and his visit was well covered by local media. A program- "Spreading Light Across the Border" (*Aman Ki Roshni*) was organized during his visit and Mayor of the city, the Inspector general of police and some other prominent personalities of city participated (Fig. 20.3). The speakers emphasized that with the help of social media the patient came to know about the center in India and he undertook this journey from Karachi to Kota. His visit to India was a unique case of human trust and empathy that knows no boundaries, neither political, nor religious. When it comes to

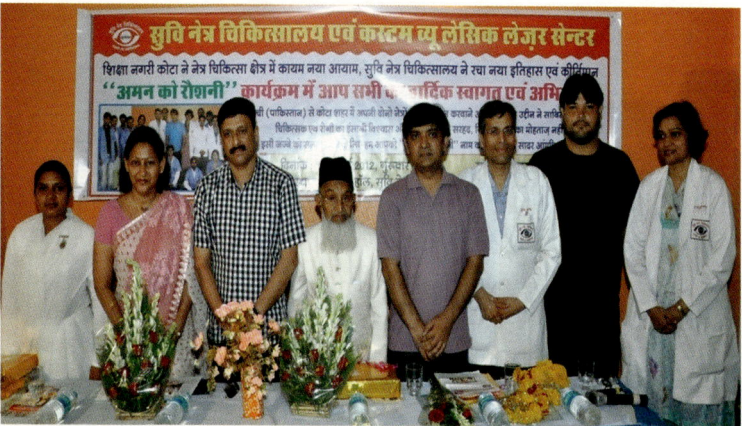

Fig. 20.3: *A program, Spreading Light Across the Border (Aman Ki Roshni), was organized during the patient's visit, in which the mayor of Kota, the Inspector General of Police, and other prominent personalities of the city participated. Left to right: Brahakumari Divisha, Mayor Dr Ratna Jain, Mr Amrit Kalash (IG Police), Mr Shahar Kazi Anwar Ahmed, Mr Fahim Uddin, Dr Suresh K Pandey, Mr Tauqeer Bokhari, and Dr Vidushi Sharma*

people to people interaction, Indians and Pakistanis have always been very warm to each other and this was just another reinforcement of the need for the two neighbors to live like friendly neighbors.

Conclusion

Social media has taken over our lives and has tremendous potential to be used as a networking tool to promote medical tourism. It provides us all a great opportunity to reach a wider audience, and eye surgery is especially suited for the sharing of surgical techniques and tips. These sites may prove to be just what the doctor ordered to bring about greater interaction and trust among people otherwise separated by manmade borders.

21 Doctors in the Society, Medical Professionalism in the Changing World and Future of Medical: Ophthalmic Practice

Vidushi Sharma, Suresh K Pandey

India's health system is undergoing enormous change. The entry of multiple health providers, the wish for more equal engagement between patients and professionals, and the ever-greater contribution of science to advances in clinical practice all demand a clear statement of medicine's unifying purpose and doctors' common values.

Medical professionalism can essentially be defined as a set of values, behaviors, and relationships. Specifically, this includes integrity, compassion, altruism, continuous improvement, excellence, and working in partnership with members of the wider health care team. Medicine bridges the gap between science and society. The application of scientific knowledge to human health is a crucial aspect of clinical practice. Doctors are one important agent through which that scientific understanding is expressed. But medicine is more than the sum of our knowledge about disease. Medicine concerns the experiences, feelings, and interpretations of human beings in often extraordinary moments of fear, anxiety, and doubt. In this extremely vulnerable position, it is medical professionalism that underpins the trust the public has in doctors.

What is medical professionalism and does it matter to patients? Although evidence is lacking that more robust professionalism will inevitably lead to better health outcomes, patients certainly understand the meaning of poor professionalism and associate it with poor medical care. The public is well aware that an absence of professionalism is harmful to their interests. The values that doctors embrace set a standard for what patients expect from their medical practitioners. The practice of medicine is distinguished by the need for judgment in the face of uncertainty. Doctors take responsibility for these judgments and their consequences. A doctor's up-to-date knowledge and skill provide the explicit scientific and often tacit experiential basis for such judgments. But because so much of medicine's unpredictability calls for wisdom as well as technical ability, doctors are vulnerable to the charge that their decisions are neither transparent nor accountable. In an age where deference is dead and league tables are the norm, doctors must be clearer about what they do, and how and why they do it.

Future of Ophthalmic Practice and Advances in the Field of Ophthalmology

Younger ophthalmologists will be more diverse demographically than their predecessors, and as a consequence, their world views and career expectations will differ greatly from those of older physicians. It will be important to recognize the different expectations of younger ophthalmologists, particularly in terms of communication and training. Because younger ophthalmologists have lived in an age of instant access, they tend to communicate and collaborate 24 hours a day via social networking sites such as Facebook and LinkedIn and specialized sites such as the American Academy of Ophthalmology, All India Ophthalmological Society, professional networking Web site, all at the convenience of the individual.

1. **Mobile diagnostic and communication tools**: EyeNetra, a Boston-based start-up, is developing *a low-cost application* designed to replace a $5,000 auto-refractor, and in September, researchers at Massachusetts Eye and Ear developed *a simple technique of fundus (retinal) photography* using an iPhone and an inexpensive application (Fundus cameras can today cost from tens to hundreds of thousands of dollars). This same month, *a surgeon wearing Google Glass performed the world's first surgery*, and as *this new video* suggests, the potential for Google Glass and other "virtual reality augmentation tools" to transform how future

ophthalmologists will be trained in the near future could be immense. Furthermore, as online educational and professional networking platforms such as *EyeTube.net* and *EyeRounds.org* begin uploading "augmented" videos practicing ophthalmologists will also be able to improve their surgical skills. (As impressive as Google Glass is as a technology, it would not stop developing. In fact, researchers in South Korea are already attempting to put "Google Glass into a contact lens.")

2. **Predictive analytics/big data:** Sloan-Kettering, one of the world's leading cancer centers, recently "hired" Watson, IBM's powerful supercomputer, *to help diagnose cancer faster*, more affordably and more accurately. In the near future, similar tools may help diagnose patients for various eye-related ailments. "Big Data" and predictive analytics may also help identify patients most at risk for not taking their medication properly—a problem estimated to cost the US health care system $300 billion a year. Once identified, however, ophthalmologists and other health care professionals will be able to take targeted action to help these at-risk individuals better adhere to their drug regiments.

3. **Pharmaceutical advances:** It has been estimated there are upwards of 500 eye-related pharmaceutical clinical trials currently under review. Many of these treatments will ultimately prove ineffective but if just a small percentage are successful they could be "game changers." Pharmaceutical solutions for presbyopia, dry-eye and myopia are real possibilities.

4. **Robotics:** Femtosecond laser surgery for the removal of cataracts is already here. The technology will only become better and more affordable in the future. As it does, robotics may soon be used in vitreoretinal surgery and various other procedures. Startling advances by entrepreneurial ophthalmologists using open-source methodologies and off-the-shelf technology to create sophisticated, low-cost surgical robots such as *Raven* may even point to an affordable robotic future. Longer term, advances in micro-

surgical devices point toward a bolder—and far less invasive—future for eye surgery.

5. **Genomics:** The cost of sequencing the human genome is plummeting. As it does, society will come to a better understanding of the roles various genes play in the development of diseases such as diabetes and retinal degeneration. This new understanding may lead to earlier and better treatment of eye-related ailments like diabetic retinopathy and retinitis pigmentosa.

6. **Retinal prosthetics:** In July 2013, The Food and Drug Administration (FDA) approved the use of *Argus II*, a bionic eye; and in September, European regulators approved the use of *the Atlas IMS*—the first fully implantable, wirelessly controlled retinal prosthetic. At the present time both devices cost approximately $1,00,000 and allow patients with retinitis pigmentosa to see in black-and-white. In the near future, as evermore electrodes are packed into the device, the technology may allow the users—including those suffering from age-related macular degeneration—to see more clearly and in color.

7. **Regenerative medicine:** The first successful *transplant of a biosynthetic cornea* occurred in 2010. Since that time, breakthroughs in biotechnology, material science and 3D printing have accelerated the field, and in the not-too-distant future, biosynthetic corneas could help restore sight to the vast number of people who are currently waiting for a donated human cornea for transplantation.

8. **Nanotechnology:** Researchers at the University of Dayton Research Institute recently created *"fuzzy fiber" carbon nanotubes*. This could be a significant breakthrough for the treatment of glaucoma because the "fuzzy fibers" are biocompatible and can help prevent the build-up of fibroblasts. Other breakthroughs in nanotechnology include using nanoparticles for gene therapy—such as this *one* for the treatment of macular degeneration—and are quite exciting.

9. **Stem cell advances:** Earlier this year, the company advanced cell technology *announced an innovative stem cell*

treatment it had developed had corrected the eyesight of an individual with 20/400 vision to 20/40. The company is equally excited about the possibility that stem cells can soon be used to treat Stargardt's macular dystrophy.

10. **Neuroscience advances:** In August, researchers at MIT and the Max Planck institute *announced they had mapped the 950 neurons in the retina of a mouse*. It is only a matter of time before the neurons in the human retina are similarly mapped. When this happens ophthalmologists under-standing of photoreceptors, horizontal cells, bipolar cells, amacrine cells and ganglion cells may lead to a new and deeper understanding of the human eye.

Violence and Aggressions Against Doctors: How to Avoid Confronting Situations?

Vidushi Sharma, Suresh K Pandey

In today's world, sadly doctors do not hold the same place of respect and there is a steadily declining mutual trust and erosion of the doctor patient relationship. While patients often complain that doctors are proud, indifferent, do not give them expected care, take hefty fees, are dominating and confuse them with a lot of medical jargon; doctors are also bitter about the increasingly aggressive attitude of patients, who are willing to fight at the drop of a hat, do not respect doctors or

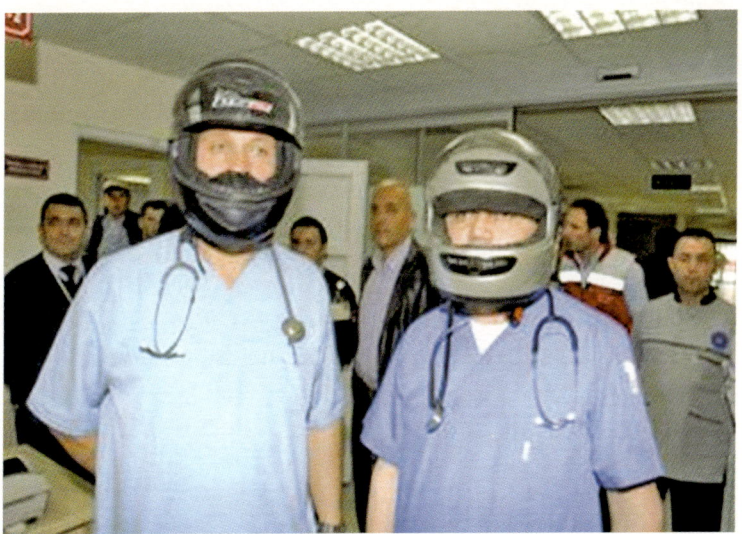

Fig. 22.1: *Doctors in Turkey with helmet to protest against violence*

their work, always blame doctors for everything without understanding the disease and its consequences. This scenario is not good for society at all as hospitals and clinics are supposed to be safe havens for the treatment and care of the sick and diseased, and we cannot afford to let them turn into battlegrounds.

In this video, the authors discuss the extent of problem? Why does it occur? What can be done? To minimize aggressions and violence against doctors.

Violence against doctors is becoming global phenomenon. Of late incidence of violence against doctors has increased. Very often we hear doctors being molested, thrashed and abused by lay public for a trivial fault, or no fault of theirs. At least in one instance, a doctor was shot dead by angry relatives. Among doctors, psychiatrists and emergency medicine physicians are believed to be at highest risk of aggression and violence. This is most likely explained by a combination of clinical and environmental factors. For example, physician inexperience, urban locale, and patient characteristics such as intoxication, acute psychosis or delirium, and drug-seeking behavior have all been described in the psychiatric and emergency medicine literature as risk factors for aggression and violence. Because these factors also exist in practice settings, physical safety is an important and valid concern.

How to Prevent Aggression and Violence Against Doctors?

1. The most important step is to restrict entry of public. At no stage hordes of relatives should be allowed at the patient's bedside. Entry should be strictly by passes and this must be implemented through good security, preferably by ex-army personnel.

2. Security guards must be placed inside the hospital at sensitive areas like ICU, operation theatre and casualty.

3. Much needs to be done to improve doctor—patient relationship. This must begin by the doctor informing the relative of what is going on. As the patient is being investigated diagnosis need not be given out. There should be no hyper bole nor understatements. Under no circumstances must the previous hospital or referring doctor be criticized.

Words such as 'You have come too late' must not be used. This puts the blame on the patient. Who then retaliates by criticizing doctors. In desperate situations patients must be given a choice of calling another doctor (second opinion) if they feel so. The suggestions of organ donation must only be made in brain death. When the prognosis is serious the senior doctors must talk to the relatives. Security must be provided to the doctors at all times and at all places when they are at work.

4. The medical association has taken up with the Government the need to make violence against doctors a nonbailable offence. Unfortunately the law has not implemented during many instances.